P9-DUP-375

Movement Therapy in Hemiplegia

with a Foreword by HELEN J. HISLOP, Ph.D.

drawings by PHILLIP CARSON

Movement Therapy in Hemiplegia

A Neurophysiological Approach

With 139 Illustrations

SIGNE BRUNNSTROM, M.A.

Graduate, Royal Gymnastic Central
Institute, Stockholm, Sweden;
Instructor in Physical Therapy,
College of Physicians & Surgeons,
Columbia University, New York City;
Educational Consultant,
New York State Rehabilitation Hospital,
West Haverstraw, New York

MEDICAL DEPARTMENT
HARPER & ROW, PUBLISHERS
HAGERSTOWN, MARYLAND
NEW YORK, SAN FRANCISCO, LONDON

MOVEMENT THERAPY IN HEMIPLEGIA:
A NEUROPHYSIOLOGICAL APPROACH

First Edition

LIBRARY OF CONGRESS CATALOG
CARD NUMBER: 70-106334

Contents

Foreword

The pursuit of knowledge is a measure of the compleat clinician. Nowhere in the profession of physical therapy is this better exemplified than by the author of this book. For here, Miss Brunnstrom summarizes a lifetime of observation, experimentation, success, and failure in the physical therapy management of the patient with hemiplegia.

She has endeavored to present a basic text which will assist the clinician and the student in appreciating and managing the tremendous complexities that arise in the classic stroke syndrome. Her approach is of her own conception and in addition to her own unique contributions, she interweaves a wealth of information from reliable sources in physiology, neurology, and other clinical sciences.

The aim of this book is the improvement of patient care. It should achieve its purpose for this is the first comprehensive text for the physical therapist on this subject. Other allied health professionals and physicians will also benefit from the information presented. Miss Brunnstrom has aimed at a unified system of management; the book is not a global discussion of the treatment of hemiplegia. It does make a significant contribution to understanding motor behavior and movement therapy for the rehabilitation of these patients by the physical therapist.

The content is developed in a sequence that is logical from a clinical viewpoint. Emphasis is given to the evaluation of the patient and then followed by succinct suggestions for treatment. The treatment procedures will be exceedingly helpful as they are clearly written and unusually complete. Also outstanding is the description of synergistic movement patterns. Case studies provide enrichment that teach by example. The appendix of abstracts is an unusual feature which will give the serious reader a direct summary of the hallmark papers which constitute the rationale for the therapeutic procedures advocated by the author.

Miss Brunnstrom's many years of experience as an inquiring clinician is the foundation of this book, for only a person with great insight into, and direct knowledge of, the problems of the patient with hemiplegia could have compiled this excellent treatise.

Downey, California

Helen J. Hislop, Ph.D.
ASSOCIATE CLINICAL PROFESSOR OF PHYSICAL THERAPY
UNIVERSITY OF SOUTHERN CALIFORNIA
SCHOOL OF MEDICINE

Preface

This book is the outcome of a special interest in patients with neuromuscular disorders, which dates from World War II. After the war, the large number of stroke patients encountered in rehabilitation clinics prompted me to turn my attention particularly to the problems of patients with hemiplegia who seemed to respond poorly to conventional training techniques. It is hoped that the techniques presented in this manual will aid the therapist, teacher, and student in their work with these patients.

Many years of study and clinical observation were required before the neurophysiological approach set forth in this book evolved. Portions of the material in the present text have been used since 1961 as part of a course dealing with the application of neurophysiological principles to human motion, a subject incorporated in the physical therapy curriculum at the College of Physicians & Surgeons, Columbia University.

In 1965, a grant from the Vocational Rehabilitation Administration, U.S. Department of Health, Education and Welfare (now The Social and Rehabilitation Service) enabled me to prepare a students' manual on the rationale and techniques of movement therapy for stroke patients. The manual was printed in Multilith form, but the supply was soon exhausted.

The favorable reception given the manual by teaching staff, students, and clinical workers alike stimulated the writing of this book. The material in the manual has been revised and enlarged, and numerous photographs have been added to illustrate the motor behavior of patients with hemiplegia and to clarify some of the training procedures discussed in the text.

Portions of the texts in Chapters 2, 4, and 5 originally appeared in *Physical Therapy, J. Amer. Phys. Ther. Ass.* 44:11, 1964; 45:17, 1965; and 46:365, 1966. Permission to use this material in the present publication is greatfully acknowledged.

The illustrations accompanying the text were derived in part from still photographs and in part from frames of motion pictures, courtesy of the following institutions:

The Burke Rehabilitation Center, White Plains, New York (Figures 2-1, 3-1 through 3-5, 3-8, and 5-2 through 5-6)

The Institute of Rehabilitation Medicine, New York (Figures 1-10, 1-13, 1-14, 3-6, 3-7, 3-9, 3-12 through 3-15, and 3-19)

The Neurological Institute, Presbyterian Medical Center, New York (Figures 1-11, 1-17, 2-2, 2-4, 2-5, 2-6, 2-9 through 2-12, 3-16 through 3-18, and 3-20).

It is hoped that the material here presented will prove of value to teachers and clinicians alike.

Carmel, N.Y.

Signe Brunnstrom

Movement
Therapy in
Hemiplegia

A prime requirement for personnel dealing with the physical rehabilitation of stroke patients is to have a basic understanding of the sensorimotor difficulties common to these patients—in fact, common to most patients with hemiplegia, whether resulting from a cerebral vascular accident or from other pathology. Without such understanding, the training methods to be described would have little meaning and might even be misunderstood. The rationale for neuromuscular therapy as practiced by the author cannot be expressed in a few words but evolves gradually from the study of scientific material and from clinical observations.

The present publication contains a picture gallery of typical sensorimotor reactions of patients with hemiplegia and should, to some extent, help the student to bridge the gap between didactic information and therapeutic applications. The illustrations and accompanying comments may also serve as an incentive for therapists to carefully observe reactions and attitudes of their patients and to attempt to interpret the meaning of their observations. Because many aspects of the motor behavior of hemiplegic patients are not well understood in terms of neurophysiology and neuropathology, continued study and research must be encouraged.

A survey of medical literature by the author yielded an abundance of material related to the motor behavior of patients with hemiplegia but few suggestions with respect to therapeutic procedures. A large number of worthwhile articles were abstracted, but if they were all included, these would fill several volumes. For the present book it became necessary to select among the most valuable scientific and clinical papers and, reluctantly, to cut the abstracts down in size. Although abstracts cannot take the place of original publications, they serve a purpose for undergraduate students and for workers in the field

Introduction

whose time does not permit as extensive reading as would be desirable. The selected and revised abstracts are found in the Appendix. The reader will find references at the end of each chapter and is advised to consult basic texts in neurophysiology.

Much reading material which the author covered substantiated clinical observations previously made; passages were also found which posed questions and required further clinical experimentation. Hypotheses purporting to explain clinical phenomena were frequently encountered in the literature, but valid scientific data to support these hypotheses are mostly missing.

Training procedures for patients with hemiplegia evolved in part from clinical findings, in part from information obtained in medical literature. The trial and error method was extensively employed and unexplained phenomena utilized as long as they appeared to have some value. Motor responses obtained in specific cases under specific conditions were often successfully evoked in other patients. Conditions under which spontaneous willed movements occurred were carefully noted, and an attempt was made to duplicate these conditions for more extensive use. Furthermore, unsolicited remarks by hemiplegic patients describing sensations accompanying successful movements furnished valuable clues for the understanding of reactions observed. Little by little, a certain insight into the patients' motor problems was gained, an insight which proved of tremendous value in dealing with individual subjects.

The nature of many sensorimotor mechanisms in experimental animals—spinal and decerebrate cats, dogs, and monkeys—was elucidated by Sherrington (1898, 1947 [first published in 1906], 1909, 1910, 1913). These mechanisms were found present also in intact animals, although they were best studied when voluntary impulses were eliminated. Much evidence is available to support the contention that afferent-efferent mechanisms which developed

during early phylogenesis have been retained also in man, although they have been depressed during the developmental period. These mechanisms have served as a basis for the evolutionary process which resulted in more voluntary and less automatic movements than those which characterize the lower species.

Magnus, a Dutch scientist and an associate of Sherrington, stressed that the central nervous system is continuously influenced by impulses from the periphery, and that these impulses may either work together to facilitate specific motor responses, or they may "compete" with each other by exerting opposite influences (Magnus, 1924, p. 49). The tonic neck and labyrinthine reflexes are examples, as they either reinforce or oppose each other (Magnus and de Kleijn, 1912).

Magnus also demonstrated by experiments on cats and dogs that the identical stimulus, such as pinching the tip of the tail of a spinal cat, may evoke opposite motor responses, depending upon the position of the responding part. These experiments exemplify the so-called Magnus-von Uexküll rule (Magnus, 1909; von Uexküll, 1905), which states that proprioceptive impulses originating in elongated muscles influence the central organ in such a way that a shunting of motor impulses into pathways leading to the elongated muscles occurs. In von Uexküll's words, quoted by Magnus (1924, p. 26), these pathways become "tuned in"—they are ready to conduct impulses. It follows that changes in joint positions in any part of the body has an effect on the central nervous system so that conduction by this or that pathway becomes facilitated or inhibited.

The effect of elongation of a muscle on its excitability was first observed by von Uexküll in experiments with the starfish. Phylogenetically, therefore, it is a very old principle, which has been retained in higher species. But Magnus hastens to point out that in the highly developed nervous system of vertebrates it is only one of many mechanisms present, and that in higher animals and under specific conditions, one shunting mechanism supersedes another; this was demonstrated in the laboratory.

That the Magnus–von Uexküll rule applies also to monkeys with intact nervous system during stimulation of the cerebral cortex was verified by Gellhorn (1948), and there is strong evidence that the rule operates also in man. Nevertheless, clinical evidence indicates that this particular rule does not necessarily apply to patients with spastic hemiplegia; in fact, in many instances elongation of a muscle appears to inhibit its response. It may be concluded that in these patients another shunting mechanism has superseded the Magnus–von Uexküll rule.

The above is intended to illustrate that categorical statements regarding facilitatory and inhibitory effects of certain procedures—such as elongation of a muscle—should not be made. Yet, techniques have been established which frequently, although not universally, enhance the initiation of a muscular contraction or reinforce a muscle group's activity in patients with hemiplegia; some of these procedures will be discussed in this book. However, the establishment of strict "cause-and-effect" dicta will be avoided because of the numerous and varying influences inherent in different situations.

Reflex movements in spinal animals, such as the flexion reflex, and the crossed extension reflex were thoroughly investigated and reported in detail by Sherrington (1910). At a later date, Hagbarth elaborated on certain aspects of Sherrington's research, conducting experiments first on cats (1952) and subsequently on human subjects (1960). Hagbarth demonstrated a striking resemblance between the flexion reflex of Sherrington and the withdrawal reflex of normal man. If the flexor synergy of the lower limb in hemiplegic patients is compared with the withdrawal reflex of normal man, it becomes evident that the movement patterns for the two responses are identical.

From this and other evidence it may be concluded that the basic limb synergies of hemiplegic patients are primitive spinal cord patterns which have been retained throughout the evolutionary process. In normal man, these spinal cord patterns are modified in a multitude of ways and their components rearranged through the influence of higher centers. But during the spastic stage of hemiplegia they retain their primitive stereotyped character.

When the influence of higher centers is temporarily or permanently interfered with, normal reflexes become exaggerated and so-called pathological reflexes appear. These same reflexes, however, were present during a certain phylogenetic period and, therefore, may be considered "normal" when in spastic hemiplegia that portion of the central nervous system which regulates motor responses has reverted to an earlier developmental stage (Jackson, 1884, Fay, 1946, 1955).

In spastic hemiplegia, many different types of afferent impulses, including those originating in the neck, in the lumbar region, and in the labyrinths, exert a marked influence on motor responses. The advisability of deliberately utilizing such afferent impulses to initiate movements which the patient is unable to produce voluntarily, or to inhibit undesired muscular responses, may be challenged by some workers in the field. It is argued that no pathological responses should be employed in training, for fear that by repeated use the efferent pathways employed by these responses become too readily available at the expense of normal pathways. According to these views, the patient must not be allowed to use the basic limb synergies of flexion and extension, nor must the effect of the tonic neck reflex and other attitudinal reflexes be evoked to facilitate or inhibit movement, but attempts must be made from the beginning to develop normal motor responses.

The author has come to the opposite conclusion, namely, that during the early recovery stages the hemiplegic patient should be aided and encouraged to gain control of the basic limb synergies, and that for such purposes selected afferent stimuli of proprioceptive and exteroceptive origin are justified and advantageous. Once the limb synergies can be performed—not necessarily full range at all joints—a modification of the synergies begins to bring out movement combinations which deviate from the synergies. Far from preventing further improvement, the synergies appear to constitute a necessary intermediate stage for further recovery. Data collected by Twitchell support the view that the gross movement synergies of flexion and extension always precede the restoration of advanced motor function following hemiplegia in man (Twitchell, 1951).

Twitchell (1951) points out that the sequence of motor recovery following hemiplegia constitutes a reversal of the disintegration of motor function observed by Denny-Brown (1950) in patients with progressive cerebral lesions of the frontal lobe. The studies of these two authors thus substantiate Jackson's hypothesis of 1884 (1958), namely, that in neurological disease an "evolution in reverse" has taken place.

Neurophysiologists often apply cutaneous stimuli to evoke motor responses in experimental animals. Such stimuli have also, to a certain extent, been found effective in facilitating willed motor acts in patients with neurological motor disorders, such as hemiplegia. It is of interest, therefore, for physical therapists to become acquainted with skin stimulation studies by Hagbarth, conducted first on spinal and on decerebrate cats (1952), then on normal human subjects (1960).

Hagbarth studied the changes in action potentials of flexor and extensor motor neurons resulting from stimulation of the skin in different areas of the lower limb. He approached the problem in a number of ways. For example, in animals he determined the influence of a "conditioning stimulus" of cutaneous origin on monosynaptic test reflexes. The resulting action potentials were recorded from efferent spinal root fibers leading to flexor and extensor muscles. In the human subjects, electrical stimuli causing a burning sensation were applied and the effects recorded by electromyography.

The results of the various studies indicate that in man as in animal, not only are flexor motor neurons excited and extensor motor neurons inhibited from most skin areas of the lower limb (as when Sherrington's flexor reflex is evoked), but skin stimulation in specific areas causes excitation of extensor motor neurons and inhibition of flexor motor neurons. In man, extensor motor neurons were excited from skin areas overlying the extensor muscles (gluteus maximus, knee extensors, calf muscles), but the effect was a *local* one and did not spread to other extensor muscles. For example, stimulation of the gluteal region resulted in discharge from the gluteus maximus muscle, but such stimulation had an *inhibitory* effect on the vastus medialis, gastrocnemius, and soleus muscles.

Hagbarth also extensively investigated the effects of various types of cutaneous stimuli. For example, his studies showed that more marked reflex effects were obtained from nociceptive and tactile and pressure end-organs than from temperature end-organs.

Judging from these studies, it would seem as though skin stimulation would be particularly applicable for local reinforcement of flexor or extensor muscles or muscle groups. This technique thus differs from reinforcement by *resistance* (proprioceptive stimulation), which commonly causes a spread of motor impulses to related muscles of a movement pattern.

Clinical experience indicates that cutaneous stimulation over *joints*, such as over the dorsum of the interphalangeal joints of the fingers, is effective in exciting extensor muscles acting over these joints while simultaneously inhibiting the antagonistic flexor muscles.

The extreme importance of sensory impulses for voluntary movement was elucidated by Mott and Sherrington (1895). In monkeys, a complete sensory denervation of a limb (upper or lower) by section of the corresponding posterior roots of spinal nerves abolished all voluntary movement. Certain automatic motor reactions were observed, but for practical purposes the limb was useless. The impairment of motor function was permanent and proved much more severe than the motor deficit resulting from ablation of a limb area in the motor cortex. Yet, on cortical stimulation, movements of the useless limb were readily evoked, indicating that the motor pathways were intact. The conclusion was that for the execution of voluntary movements the entire sensory pathway from the periphery to the cortex must be functioning.

The devastating effect of section of sensory roots occurred only when the denervation was complete; if one or the other root was spared, the motor deficit was much less. It was also demonstrated that the retainment of cutaneous sensation was more important for motor acts than the retainment of sensation originating in the muscles, and this applied in particular to the function of the hand.

In later years, Lassek (1953) and Twitchell (1954) repeated some of the above experiments. The results obtained by Mott and Sherrington were confirmed and further light was shed on the role of sensory impulses in motor acts.

The preceding pages introduce the student to the assumed rationale underlying some of the training techniques that are discussed in this book (mainly in Chapters 3 and 5). The author has refrained from discussing much recent research in neurophysiology, such as the function of the muscle spindle, its spinal and supraspinal connections. The omissions are made purposely, partly because of the complicated functions of these structures, not yet fully understood; partly because the author wishes to avoid drawing hasty conclusions in attempting to relate research findings to clinical situations. The reader is referred to Shambes' excellent review of the function of the muscle spindle which summarizes up-to-date information on the subject; it includes an extensive reference list which invites to further study (Shambes, 1968).

REFERENCES

DENNY-BROWN, D. Disintegration of motor function resulting from cerebral lesion. *J. Nerv. Ment. Dis.* 112:1, 1950.

FAY, T. Observations on the rehabilitation of movement in cerebral palsy problems. *W. Virginia Med. J.* 42:77, 1946.

FAY, T. The origin of human movement. *Amer. J. Psychiat.* 3:644, 1955.

GELLHORN, E. The influence of alterations in posture of the limbs on cortically induced movements. *Brain* 71:26, 1948.

HAGBARTH, K. E. Excitatory and inhibitory skin areas for flexor and extensor motoneurones. *Acta physiol. scand.* 26, Suppl. 94, 1952.

HAGBARTH, K. E. Spinal withdrawal reflexes in human lower limb. *J. Neurol., Neurosurg., Psychiat.* 23:222, 1960.

JACKSON, J. H. "Evolution and Dissolution of the Nervous System" (1884), in *Selected Writings of John Hughlings Jackson,* ed. by J. Taylor. New York, Basic Books, 1958, pp. 45–75.

LASSEK, A. M. Inactivation of voluntary motor function following rhizotomy. *J. Neuropath. Exper. Neurol.* 12:83, 1953.

MAGNUS, R. Zur Regelung der Bewegungen durch das Zentralnervensystem, I and II. *Pflüger Arch. Physiol.* 130:219, and 130:253, 1909.

MAGNUS, R. *Körperstellung.* Berlin, Springer, 1924, pp. 26, 49.

MAGNUS, R., and DE KLEIJN, A. Die Abhängigkeit des Tonus der Extremitätenmuskeln von der Kopfstellung. *Pflüger Arch. Physiol.* 145:455, 1912.

MOTT, F. W., and SHERRINGTON, C. S. Experiments upon the influence of sensory nerves upon movement and nutrition of the limbs. *Proc. Roy. Soc.* (London) 57:481, 1895.

SHAMBES, G. M. Influence of the muscle spindle on posture and movement. *J. Amer. Phys. Ther. Ass.* 48:1094, 1968.

SHERRINGTON, C. S., Decerebrate rigidity and reflex coordination of movement. *J. Physiol.* *22*:319, 1898.

SHERRINGTON, C. S. On plastic tonus and proprioceptive reflexes. *Quart. J. Exp. Physiol.* *2*:109, 1909.

SHERRINGTON, C. S. Flexion reflex of the limb, crossed extension reflex and reflex stepping in standing. *J. Physiol.* *40*:28, 1910.

SHERRINGTON, C. S. Reflex inhibition as a factor in the coordination of movements and postures. *Quart. J. Exper. Physiol.* *6*:251, 1913.

SHERRINGTON, C. S. *The Integrative Action of the Nervous System,* 2nd ed. New Haven, Yale Univ. Press, 1947.

TWITCHELL, T. E. The restoration of motor function following hemiplegia in man. *Brain* *74*:443, 1951.

TWITCHELL, T. E. Sensory factors in purposive movement. *J. Neurophysiol.* *17*:239, 1954.

VON UEXKÜLL, J. Studien über den Tonus II. Die Bewegungen der Schlangensterne. *Z. Biol.* *46*:1, 1905.

Persons with lesions affecting certain portions of the vascular system of the brain—mainly the areas supplied by the middle cerebral artery—exhibit motor disturbances in one half of the body; hence, the disability is referred to as hemiplegia or hemiparesis. Sensory disturbances are frequently, although not universally, present; like the motor disturbances, the sensory deficits appear in the body half that is opposite the brain lesion.

The largest number of patients with hemiplegia seen in a rehabilitation clinic are the so-called "stroke patients" who have suffered cerebral vascular accidents as a result of thrombosis, hemorrhage, embolus, or aneurysm. Hemiplegia may also be of traumatic origin or may be caused by a neoplasm. The degree of involvement as well as the differential diagnosis vary greatly among patients with hemiplegia; yet numerous common characteristics may be observed and some of these will presently be discussed. These common characteristics, however, do not exclude individual differences among patients because no two patients are exactly alike.

THE BASIC LIMB SYNERGIES

In most patients the flaccidity that follows the acute episode is sooner or later replaced by spasticity. It is during the early spastic period that the hemiplegic limb synergies make their appearance, either as reflex responses or as voluntary movements, or both. Whether evoked reflexly or performed voluntarily, the synergies are almost stereotyped. They consist either of a gross flexor movement (flexor synergy) or a gross extensor movement (extensor synergy). Variations do occur, but these are related mainly to the relative strength of the synergy components and do not indicate a change in the nature of the synergies. Neurophysio-

Motor Behavior of Adult Patients with Hemiplegia

1

7

logically, the muscles that are activated in a synergy are firmly linked together. A patient with hemiplegia is unable to recruit these same muscles for different movement combinations and cannot master individual joint movements. This is what Beevor (1903) meant when he stated that a muscle may be "paralyzed" for one movement but not for another.

The above-mentioned motor difficulties of patients with hemiparesis were well known to Hughlings Jackson, a prominent British neurologist. In his Croonian Lectures entitled *Evolution and Dissolution of the Nervous System,* delivered in 1884, (Jackson, 1958) presents a hypothesis which furnishes a neurophysiological explanation for the motor behavior of patients with hemiplegia. The phylogenetic organization of the nervous centers, he states, occurs on three levels, and this organization is recapitulated during ontogenesis. The three groups of nervous centers are integral parts of the fully developed nervous system of human adults.

The motor representation for skeletal muscles in the central nervous system are described by Jackson as follows:

The *lowest motor centers* represent all the muscles of the body in few movement combinations. They are centers for "most automatic" movements. The *middle motor centers* re-represent all the muscles of the body in more numerous combinations. They are centers for more voluntary, "less automatic" movements. The *highest motor centers* re–rerepresent the muscles of the body in "most numerous and most voluntary" combinations.

Under certain pathological circumstances, Jackson postulates, the nervous system reverts to a lower level of evolution. A *dissolution* of the nervous system, which may be expressed as *evolution in reverse,* has taken place. According to Jackson, the common type of hemiplegia, caused by a lesion in the internal capsule, affects the middle motor centers. Patients so afflicted, therefore, must rely mainly on the lowest motor centers, which provide

for relatively automatic movements and allow few movement combinations (Jackson, 1884.)

Since Jackson's time great strides have been made in medical sciences, and neurophysiologists of today may not in every respect subscribe to his theories. Nevertheless, Jackson's theories give a well-formulated, although rather elementary, explanation of the neuropathology of patients with hemiplegia and express in a simple manner the typical motor characteristics of these patients.

Severely involved patients may remain indefinitely in the stage that allows for few movement combinations only; that is, they may be able to utilize the basic limb synergies or some of their components, but may be unable to control other movement patterns. Less severely involved patients may recover sufficiently to utilize the "middle motor centers" so that more movement combinations become available. Full motor recovery requires normal functioning of the "middle motor centers." (The highest centers are usually not involved in hemiplegia.)

Each of the four limb synergies—two for the upper, two for the lower limb—incorporate specific movement components, regardless of whether the synergy is elicited reflexly or performed voluntarily by the patient. However, voluntary impulses, if interacting with impulses of reflex origin, may considerably change the outcome.

FLEXOR SYNERGY OF UPPER LIMB

If complete range of all components materializes, this synergy consists of the following:

1. Flexion of the elbow to an acute angle
2. Full-range supination of the forearm
3. Abduction of the shoulder to 90 degrees
4. External rotation of the shoulder
5. Retraction and/or elevation of the shoulder girdle

This synergy evoked as an associated reaction is illustrated in Figure 1-1A. In

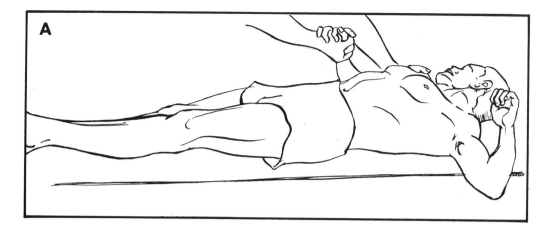

FIGURE 1-1. Flexor synergy of the upper limb in 39-year-old patient with left-sided hemiparesis of traumatic origin, 9 weeks following injury. *A.* Flexor synergy evoked as an associated reaction by resistance to elbow flexion on the normal side. The tonic neck reflex facilitates the flexor synergy. *B.* Flexor synergy performed voluntarily, facilitated by the tonic neck reflex.

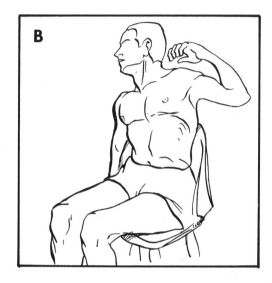

Figure 1-1*B*, the synergy is performed semivoluntarily.

EXTENSOR SYNERGY OF UPPER LIMB

The extensor synergy (when complete) has the following components:

1. Extension of the elbow, complete range
2. Full-range pronation of the forearm
3. Adduction of the arm in front of the body
4. Internal rotation of the arm
5. Fixation of the shoulder girdle in a somewhat protracted position

Figure 1-2 illustrates this synergy, evoked as an associate reaction and performed semivoluntarily.

The behavior of wrist and fingers varies considerably in individuals. Flexion of wrist and fingers commonly accompanies the flexor synergy; extension of the wrist with fist closure often appears with the extensor synergy; but these are by no means universal rules. Finger extension is not seen in either synergy; it does not gen-

erally appear until the influence of the synergies is on the decline.

FLEXOR SYNERGY OF LOWER LIMB

The components are as follows:

1. Dorsiflexion of the toes
2. Dorsiflexion and inversion of the ankle
3. Flexion of the knee to about 90 degrees
4. Flexion of the hip
5. Abduction and external rotation of the hip

This synergy evoked as an associated reaction is seen in Figure 1-3. The patient could also perform the movement voluntarily.

EXTENSOR SYNERGY OF LOWER LIMB

The components are:

1. Plantar flexion of the toes (inconsistent, great toe may extend)
2. Plantar flexion and inversion of the ankle
3. Extension of the knee
4. Extension of the hip
5. Abduction and internal rotation of the hip

This synergy evoked as an associated reaction is seen in Figure 1-4. Because hip and knee were already extended, the synergy manifested itself as plantar flexion of the ankle with inversion, tensing of the quadriceps muscles, adduction and internal rotation of the hip

REVERSAL OF MOVEMENT DIRECTIONS

The joint movements of the extensor synergy occur in the opposite direction from those of the flexor synergy. This is true not only for flexor and extensor components but also for the other components. Abduction and external rotation at shoulder and hip accompany the flexor synergies, adduction and internal rotation the extensor synergies. Dorsiflexion of the ankle is an integral part of the flexor synergy, plantar flexion of the extensor synergy. However, inversion of the ankle accompanies both the flexor and the extensor synergies. Eversion of the ankle has never been seen by this author in either synergy.

In the upper limb, extension of the wrist may be considered a component of the extensor synergy and flexion of the wrist a component of the flexor synergy, but variations do occur and will be discussed later.

COMPARATIVE STRENGTH OF SYNERGY COMPONENTS

Flexor Synergy, Upper Limb

Elbow flexion is usually the strongest component of the flexor synergy and the first one to appear following a cerebral vascular accident. Abduction and external rotation of the shoulder are often weak components. They may appear later during the recovery period or remain permanently weak so that the patient never learns to abduct the arm full range, which for the flexor synergy is 90 degrees. When the abduction and external rotation components are weak, retraction of the arm at the shoulder (hyperextension of the arm) generally appears, as seen in Figures 1-5 and 1-6.

When attempting to move the arm, the patient in Figure 1-5 elevated the shoulder girdle, combined mild abduction of the shoulder with hyperextension, flexed the elbow to an acute angle, and supinated the forearm complete range. The wrist and the fingers flexed part range. Prior to the initiation of the movement, the forearm rested in the lap in a pronated position and the fingers were relaxed in a comfortably extended position.

The flexor synergy displayed by the patient in Figure 1-6 has a similar feature, but the synergy as a whole is weaker. Even with the greatest effort the patient was unable to flex the elbow much beyond 90 degrees; the forearm supinated only half range, and no abduction or external rotation came through.

Neurophysiologically, there is a close link between the flexor muscles of the elbow and the supinators of the forearm, hence the movement of flexion of the elbow and supination of the forearm tend to occur together, as illustrated in Figures 1-5 and 1-6. But if pronator spasticity is marked, which is frequently the case when the hemiparetic condition is of longer standing, the forearm may remain pronated during the performance of the flexor synergy, as in Figure 1-7. The patient, a 33-year-old woman, had suffered a cerebral vascular accident at the age of 25 following childbirth. The pronator muscles as well as the flexor muscles of the wrist were markedly spastic.

Figure 1-8 illustrates a flexor synergy performed by a 48-year-old patient whose

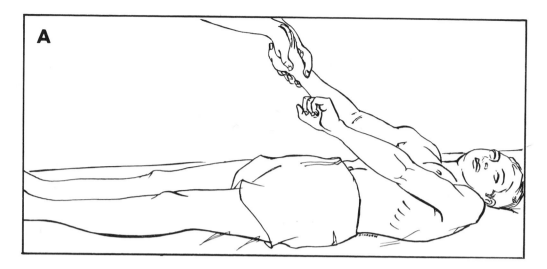

A

FIGURE 1-2. Extensor synergy of the upper limb in 39-year-old patient with left-sided hemiparesis of traumatic origin, 9 weeks following injury. *A.* Extensor synergy evoked as an associated reaction by resistance to a push on the normal side. *B.* Semivoluntary performance of the extensor synergy. Stabilization of the upper limb on the normal side and rotation of the head were required to enable the patient to carry out extension.

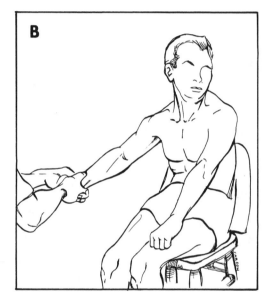

B

cerebral vascular accident had occurred five years earlier. Spasticity was marked throughout the upper limb, notably so in the pronators of the forearm, which muscles kept the forearm pronated as the shoulder abducted. External rotation of the shoulder could not be performed. In this patient, wrist extension occurred in the flexor synergy, which may be interpreted as resulting from the commonly observed linkage between the pronators of the forearm and the extensor muscles of the wrist.

Figure 1-9 shows a patient who performed the flexor synergy with complete range of external rotation at the shoulder but who was unable to abduct full range. It was suggested to the patient that he rotate the head toward the right in the hope that the tonic neck reflex would aid in increasing the range of abduction. However, no observable facilitation resulted from head rotation.

There appears to be a rather strong association between the external rotators of the shoulder and the supinators of the forearm and also between the internal rotators of the shoulder and the pronators of the forearm. In Figure 1-9 the external rotators of the shoulder and the supinators of the forearm are activated as part of the flexor synergy, there being no marked spasticity in the antagonistic muscles. But in Figure 1-8, where pronator tension is strong, no external rotation materializes. It may be assumed that this relationship has a functional basis; in most positions of the arm, turning the palm up and down is accomplished by team work between the supinators of the forearm and the external

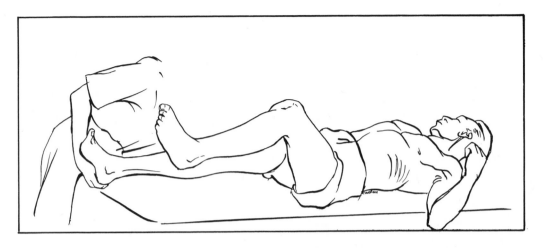

rotators of the shoulder, and by the pronators of the forearm and the internal rotators of the shoulder, respectively.

Extensor Synergy, Upper Limb

By far the strongest component of the extensor synergy is the pectoralis major muscle, the muscle mainly responsible for internal rotation and adduction of the arm in front of the body. When flaccidity subsides and spasticity begins to develop, the pectoralis major muscle is the first component of the extensor synergy to display tension and the first one to respond to voluntary effort. Pronator tension is likely to appear next, although ability to pronate the forearm voluntarily does not develop until later.

FIGURE 1-3. Flexor synergy of the affected lower limb evoked as an associated reaction by resistance to plantar flexion of the ankle on the healthy side. Same patient as in Figures 1-1 and 1-2.

In patients who exhibit marked spasticity in the upper limb, the involuntary arm posture seen in Figures 1-10A and 1-10B is commonly observed in erect standing and walking. Because of the frequency of this arm posture among patients with hemiplegia it has been called "the typical arm posture in hemiplegia." This attitude combines the strongest component of the flexor

FIGURE 1-4. Extensor synergy of the affected lower limb evoked as an associated reaction by resistance to dorsiflexion of the ankle on the normal side. Same patient as in Figures 1-1 to 1-3.

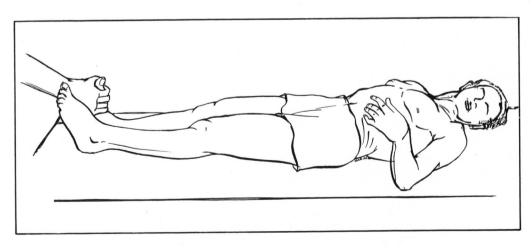

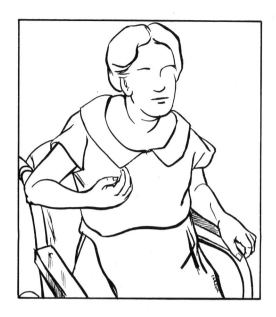

FIGURE 1-5. Flexor synergy with hyperextension at shoulder and complete range of supination of forearm.

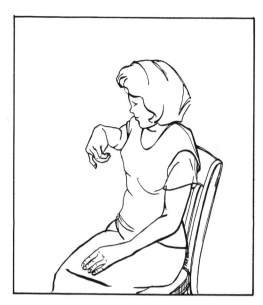

FIGURE 1-7. Flexor synergy in the presence of spasticity in the pronators of the forearm and the flexors of wrist and fingers. Hemiparesis of long standing.

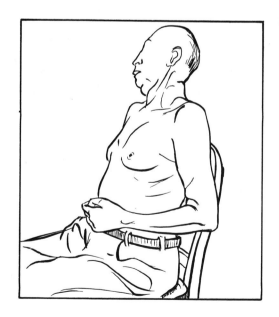

FIGURE 1-6. Flexor synergy with hyperextension at shoulder and half-range supination of forearm.

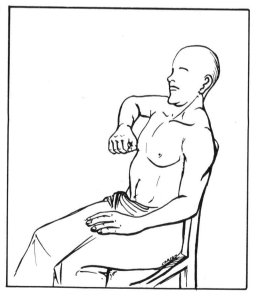

FIGURE 1-8. Flexor synergy in the presence of marked spasticity in the pronators of the forearm.

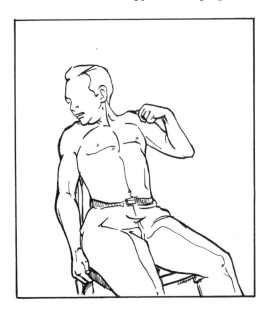

FIGURE 1-9. Flexor synergy in 38-year-old patient with left-sided hemiparesis of traumatic origin, 2½ years following injury. External rotation at shoulder and supination of forearm are complete.

synergy (elbow flexion) with the two strongest components of the extensor synergy (pronation of the forearm, adduction at the shoulder). In general, elbow extension is a weak component of the extensor synergy and appears later than the other two components. In the arm posture described, some spasticity is likely to be present in the triceps muscles, but the elbow flexors, which in the erect position are antigravity muscles, have far more tension, hence the elbow remains flexed. When initiation of elbow extension first succeeds, it does so only in conjunction with the other two extensor components.

Flexor Synergy, Lower Limb

Hip flexion appears to be the strongest component of the flexor synergy of the lower limb. It might not be very easy for the patient to initiate hip flexion in the supine position, but if the hip and the knee have first been placed in slight flexion, the hip flexor muscles often display considerable strength. The dorsiflexor mus-

cles of the ankle, once activated during hip flexion, may also have great strength if tested against resistance. The ankle muscles, seldom, if ever, are seen to initiate the flexor synergy; their activity appears to be evoked by stimuli originating in the hip flexor muscles. The movements of abduction and external rotation of the hip, which occur during flexion, do not show much strength.

Extensor Synergy, Lower Limb

The extensor synergy of the lower limb manifests itself strongly at the knee and is accompanied by plantar flexion and a variable amount of inversion of the ankle. In severely involved patients, the adductor component may be so strong that the affected limb crosses in front of the unaffected limb (Fig. 5-6 *C*). These three components—knee extension, hip adduction, and plantar flexion of the ankle with inversion—are all strong components. Internal rotation of the hip is weaker and of limited range. Hip extension appears to be a rather weak component of the extensor synergy. Weight bearing on the affected limb markedly reinforces the extensor synergy, particularly its strong components.

ATTITUDINAL OR POSTURAL REFLEXES

TONIC NECK AND LABYRINTHINE REFLEXES

The tonic neck and labyrinthine reflexes are known as "Magnus' and de Kleijn's reflexes" after two Dutch scientists who discovered the rules that govern these phenomena (Magnus and de Kleijn, 1912). The most convincing experiments of these investigators were conducted on decerebrate animals, because in such preparations no voluntary impulses disturb the reactions; but the presence of these reflexes also in intact animals was established without a doubt.

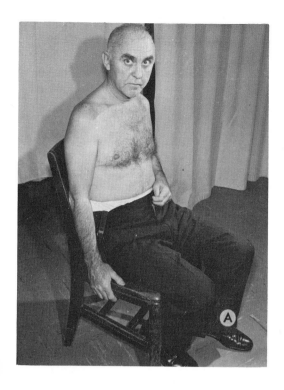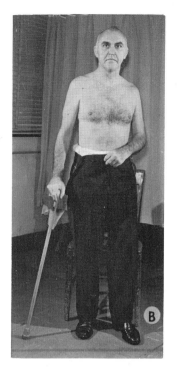

The *tonic neck reflexes* are evoked by neck movements or neck positions; they are either *symmetrical,* as in flexion and extension of the neck, or *asymmetrical,* as in rotation or side-bending of the head and neck. The symmetrical neck reflexes act identically on the limbs on the left and on the right sides; the asymmetrical neck reflexes have opposite effects on the left and on the right limbs. In each case, proprioceptive impulses originating in the cervical region affect the reflex centers in a predictable manner, as discovered by Magnus and de Kleijn.

Symmetrical Neck Reflexes

In animals, ventroflexion of the neck results in flexion of both forelimbs and extension of both hindlimbs; dorsiflexion of the neck has the opposite effect, that is, extension of both forelimbs and flexion of both hindlimbs. These two attitudes may be visualized by analyzing the events that take place when a quadruped animal creeps under a fence. First, the head is

FIGURE 1-10. Arm posture in sitting and standing, typical of patients with spastic hemiplegia. Patient, age 54, has a left-sided hemiparesis of 14 months' standing, resulting from a cerebral vascular accident. *A.* Thumb in palm of hand; spasticity present in the pronators of the forearm and in the flexors of elbow, wrist, and fingers. *B.* Arm posture much like that in sitting, but muscular tension is more marked; internal rotation at shoulder and pronation of forearm have increased. (*A* from Brunnstrom, S. Motor behavior of adult hemiplegic patients: Hints for training. *Amer. J. Occup. Ther.* 15:6, 1961.)

lowered and the forelimbs flex while the hindlimbs are still extended; then, as the animal moves forward, the head is raised and the forelimbs extend; at this time, the hindlimbs flex to permit the hind part of the body to follow.

Asymmetrical Neck Reflexes

The asymmetrical neck reflexes are governed by "flexion of the skull limbs" and "extension of the jaw limbs." When the jaw of the animal is rotated to the left, the left limbs become the "jaw limbs" and

15

extend; the right limbs become the "skull limbs" and flex. The facilitatory effect of the asymmetrical tonic neck reflex in a patient with hemiplegia is illustrated in Figures 1-1 and 1-2.

Tonic Labyrinthine Reflexes

The tonic labyrinthine reflexes are evoked by changes of the animal's head in space. When the head is in a position normal for the animal (as in quadruped posture, but with the animal held freely in the air) extensor tone in the limbs is minimal; when the animal is turned so that its belly is up, extensor tone in the limbs is maximal. The two positions are 180 degrees apart. (See Fig. 1 in Abstract 16.)

Hoff (1933) recorded the effect of tonic neck and labyrinthine reflexes on single motor units of the soleus, a "red" postural extensor muscle. When the animal's head was rotated toward the side on which the recordings were made, the rate of discharge of the single motor unit was increased, and the high rate of discharge continued as long as the head position was maintained. When the head was rotated toward the opposite side, the discharge rate diminished, followed by a cessation of electrical activity.

Tonic neck reflexes in normal infants were reported by Schaltenbrandt (1928), by Gesell and associates (1940), and by Gesell and Ames (1950). The persistence of readily demonstrable tonic neck reflexes in children several months old or older is a sign of widespread cerebral damage (Byers, 1938).

Various opinions have been expressed regarding the desirability of utilizing tonic neck reflexes for training purposes (Fay, 1946, 1955; Doman and associates, 1960), or attempting to inhibit these reflexes in children with cerebral palsy at an early date (Bobath and Bobath, 1954).

Weak attitudinal reflexes in normal adult persons were demonstrated by Ikay (1950) and by Tokizane and associates (1951). Studies by Hellebrandt and associates

(1956) and by Waterland and Hellebrandt (1964) indicate that the tonic neck reflex is utilized automatically by normal persons to reinforce voluntary effort during activities involving heavy resistance.

TONIC LUMBAR REFLEXES

The tonic lumbar reflexes were discovered by two Japanese investigators, Shimamoto and Nakajima, quoted by Tokizane and associates (1951). These reflexes are elicited by changes in the position of the upper part of the body with respect to the pelvis. Rotation, lateral bending, forward and backward bending of the upper body in relation to the pelvis were found to have specific influences on the tone of the muscles of the limbs. As an example, a rotation of the front part of the chest to the right was found to facilitate flexion of the right upper limb and extension of the right lower limb; a rotation to the left facilitated extension of the right upper limb and flexion of the right lower limb. The effects on the left side were opposite to those on the right side.

These movement combinations are employed in various athletic activities, such as throwing a ball or a javelin, and serving in tennis. If the racket is held in the right hand, the trunk is first rotated to the right, the right arm is pulled backward (flexed), and the body weight is shifted onto the right leg, which requires stabilization by extensor muscles. After the ball has been tossed up in the air and as the ball is hit, the trunk rotates toward the left, the right arm is flung forward (extends), and the body weight is shifted to the left leg while the right foot is taken off the ground (flexes). In throwing activities, the facilitating effects of the tonic neck reflexes are also utilized.

The presence of weak tonic lumbar reflexes and of neck and labyrinthine reflexes in four normal persons was demonstrated by Tokizane and associates (1951). Electromyographic recordings from flexor and extensor muscles of the upper and lower limbs showed increase and decrease of discharge rates of motor units of these muscles in accordance with the rules for the above types of reflexes. The changes in the position of the head with respect to the trunk, of the upper body with respect to the pelvis, and of the position of the head in space were passively accomplished. The neck reflexes were found to have more marked effect on the upper, the lumbar reflexes on the lower limbs. A deaf-mute person who participated in the study displayed the same effects from neck and lumbar reflexes as the normal subjects, but no effects from the labyrinths was demonstrated.

The various studies reviewed here indicate that attitudinal reflexes that are laid down in the nervous system at an early phylogenetic date are still part of the neurophysiological equipment of normal children and adults, and that, under various circumstances, their facilitating effects may still be utilized.

The attitudinal reflexes become easily demonstrable (because exaggerated) in the presence of certain types of pathology of the nervous system. Walshe describes typical and marked tonic neck reflexes acting on the limbs (elicited by passive rotation of the head) in a woman patient who, because of a brain tumor, was in a state of decerebrate rigidity (1923a). In children with cerebral palsy and in adult patients with spastic hemiplegia the attitudinal reflexes (as well as other types of reflexes) are exaggerated more often than not. Their influence may even be so strong that a patient may be able to perform voluntary flexor and extensor movements only by utilizing the facilitating effect of one or the other of these reflexes. When a conflict between the will and inhibitory reflex impulses exists, the will does not always gain supremacy.

ASSOCIATED REACTIONS

In patients with hemiparesis reflex tensing of muscles and involuntary limb movement are frequently observed. These responses are known as *associated reactions*. In most patients, voluntary forceful movements in other parts of the body readily elicit such reactions in the affected limbs. If the voluntary effort is strong and of some duration, *associated movements* may appear, involving several or all of the joints of the affected limb or limbs. When the associated movement comes to a halt, either at full range or short of full range, muscular tension continues, and the affected limb is held in a rigid posture until the stimulus that evoked the reaction ceases. Then muscular tension in the limb gradually diminishes.

Riddoch and Buzzard (1921) defined associated reactions as "automatic activities which fix or alter the posture of a part or parts when some other part of the body is brought into action by either voluntary effort or reflex stimulation."

In the experience of this author, associated movements are more commonly elicited when spasticity is present than when the condition is essentially flaccid. Yet, for some unexplained reason, patients are occasionally found who exhibit vivid associated responses even though little or no spasticity can be demonstrated in the responding limb or limbs. Such an associated reaction in a patient with left-sided hemiparesis is shown in Figure 1-11.

EXAMPLES OF ASSOCIATED REACTIONS

Case 1

The patient, a 35-year-old male, developed a left-sided hemiparesis as a result of a thrombosis of the right middle cerebral artery. Several months prior to the cerebral vascular accident, repeated minor episodes of sensory and motor deficit had occurred. The last attack was sudden, and the patient fell to the floor. He was admitted to the hospital the same day.

Four weeks following the patient's hospital admission, the sensorimotor status of the left upper limb, grossly tested, was as

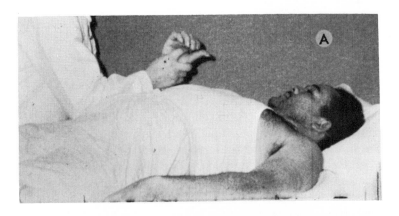

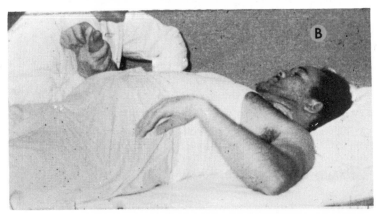

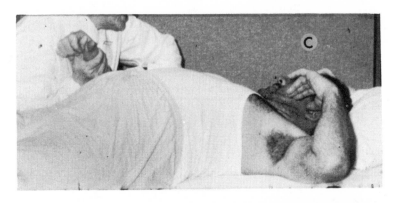

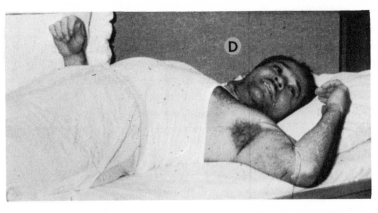

FIGURE 1-11. Associated flexor synergy evoked in the upper limb of a patient with left-sided flaccid hemiparesis. (Frames from a motion picture.) *A.* Resistance to elbow extension on the normal side has no immediate effect on the left arm. *B.* With increased effort, an associated reaction appears in the left arm, that is, the elbow flexes. *C.* As the effort is sustained, elbow flexion continues, the shoulder abducts and externally rotates, and the forearm supinates. *D.* The stimulus has been discontinued; the arm remains above the head. The patient had been unaware of the associated reaction and was pleased to discover that the arm had moved.

follows: position sense was totally absent; gross passive movements of the affected limb were vaguely felt, but the patient could not distinguish the direction of a movement, neither at proximal nor at distal joints. Fingertip recognition was absent. The limb felt heavy when moved passively, and no muscular resistance to passive motions was detected. The patient could not voluntarily initiate any arm movements.

The patient attended the physical therapy clinic regularly, but for several weeks there was no improvement in the upper limb. About 2 months following the acute episode, heavy resistance was applied on the normal side, first to elbow flexion, then to elbow extension. Surprisingly, a vivid associated flexor synergy appeared on the affected side (Fig. 1-11).

During this experiment, the patient had been looking toward the therapist and had been focusing his attention on forcefully extending the elbow on that side. He therefore had not seen the movement of the affected arm, nor had he felt it, because passive motion sense of the affected upper limb was absent. (Following the discovery of the associated movement of the affected upper limb, this reaction was utilized during training sessions, as described in Chapter 3.)

This case illustrates the following:

1. An associated movement may be evoked in a limb which is essentially flaccid and over which its owner has no control. (Latent spasticity may be present.)
2. In the upper limb, a flexor response is more easily evoked than an extensor response. (The investigator was unable to evoke extension.)
3. Repeated stimuli may be required to evoke a response. (The first few trials met with no success.)
4. When the reaction finally materialized, a full-range flexor synergy appeared.
5. Tension in the muscles of the affected

limb decreased rapidly after cessation of the stimulus that had evoked the associated reaction.

Case 2

Figure 1-12 illustrates associated reactions in a patient with moderate spasticity of the upper limb. The patient, age 49, had a right-sided hemiparesis; the acute episode had occurred four years earlier. He performed both the flexor and the extensor synergies voluntarily but had not mastered other movement combinations.

Figure 1-12 *A* and *B* shows that voluntary movements were markedly influenced by the limb synergies. When the patient attempted to raise the arms laterally to a horizontal position, the left arm performed as requested, but on the right side a flexor synergy developed (*A*). The patient was unable to keep the right elbow extended when abducting the shoulder because of the strong linkage between the various components of the flexor synergy. When the patient was asked to reach overhead, the affected arm was only raised slightly higher than before (*B*).

Thereafter, the patient was told that the strength of the normal hand was to be tested. As he forcefully clenched the dynamometer, an associated flexor response appeared on the affected side (Fig. 1-12*C*), and this response closely resembled the voluntary abduction movement.

Next the patient kept his head rotated toward the unaffected side while retesting his grip strength. The associated movement appeared as before, but this time external rotation of the shoulder was added, and the final position was higher than before (Fig. 1-12*D*). The altered head position apparently had reinforced the response.

After the patient had clenched the dynamometer as forcefully as he could with the head rotated to the left, he looked down to read the result on the dynamometer (Fig.

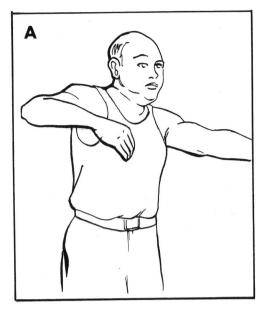

A

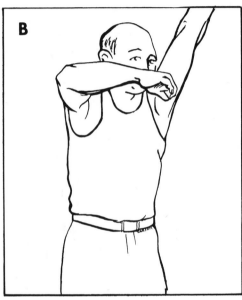

B

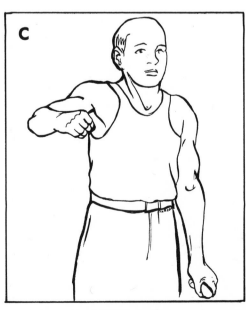

C

1-12E). The illustration suggests that the muscular tension in the arm was slow in disappearing, and that the patient was unaware of the slow downward movement of the limb.

The test was now repeated while the patient kept his head rotated toward the affected side. The right arm first responded with flexion of the elbow and abduction of the shoulder (Fig. 1-12F), then the movement changed its direction and the arm moved slowly into the paths of the extensor synergy (Fig. 1-12G). This movement reversal may be interpreted as a result of the effect of the tonic neck reflex.

We learn the following from this case:

1. Associated movements may occur in the affected limb in the presence of spasticity and when the patient has a degree of voluntary control of limb movements.
2. When the basic movement synergies dominate the behavior, a patient may be unable, even with greatest effort, to overcome the synergy influence.
3. The flexor synergy of the upper limb is easier to elicit than the extensor synergy; flexion appeared when the head was in a neutral position.
4. The asymmetrical tonic neck reflex influences the outcome of the associated movement.
5. Associated movements may be present years after the onset of hemiplegia, in this case four years following the acute episode.

FIGURE 1-12. A 49-year-old patient with right-sided hemiparesis, 5 years following a cerebral vascular accident. (Drawn from frames of a motion picture.) *A.* The patient attempts to raise both arms laterally to a horizontal position. On the affected side a flexor synergy develops. The patient is unable to combine abduction of the shoulder with extension of the elbow. *B.* The patient attempts to raise both arms overhead. The range of the flexor synergy increases somewhat, but the elbow remains flexed and the arm cannot be raised much above the horizontal position. *C.* Forceful gripping of a dynamometer in the unaffected hand evokes an associated move-

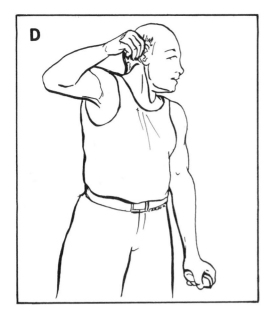

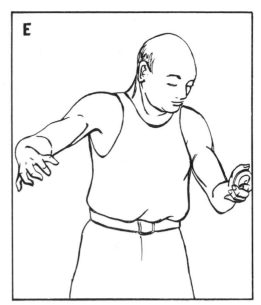

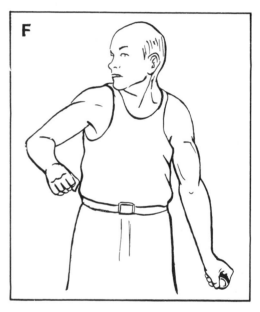

6. As long as the limb synergies are dominant, voluntary and associated movements are likely to have identical shapes, and both are manifestations of primitive movement patterns.

Case 3

A third patient who had left-sided involvement of traumatic origin had progressed to a point of near normal motor control of the proximal joints of the left arm. Little or no spasticity remained, and during willed movements no influence of the synergies was detected. Yet, he exhibited rapid and full range associated move-

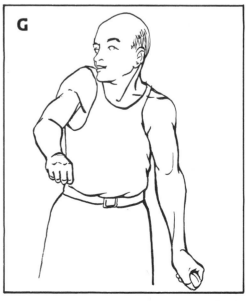

ment of the affected arm, which takes the shape of a flexor synergy. *D.* Head rotation to the left reinforces the flexor synergy which, as before, is evoked by clenching a dynamometer. External rotation of the shoulder and partial supination of the forearm have been added. *E.* Patient reads the result of the manometer test. The affected arm is slow in returning to the side of the body. The hand, previously closed, has opened up in a peculiar manner. *F* and *G.* With the head rotated toward the affected side, the patient again forcefully grips the dynamometer. In spite of the head position, the affected arm begins to flex *(F)*; with sustained effort, however, extension follows *(G).*

ments of the left upper limb, and these movements were markedly influenced by the tonic neck reflexes.

When the patient squeezed a piece of sponge rubber in the normal hand while the head was rotated toward the normal side, a typical flexor synergy developed on the affected side. If the head was rotated to the other side and the stimulus repeated, an extensor synergy appeared.

Case 3 illustrates the following:

1. Associated movements may appear in a limb after spasticity has essentially subsided.
2. Voluntary control of a large variety of arm movements does not necessarily exclude the appearance of typical associated reactions.
3. An influence of the asymmetrical tonic neck reflex may be present during advanced recovery stages.

It should be added, however, that this case is an unusual one, the exception rather than the rule. The patient had recovered normal, or near normal, control of the proximal joints, but the hand remained affected in a rather peculiar way. When the arm was in the overhead position, he closed and opened the affected hand full range without difficulty. When the arm was lowered, he could still make a fist but he could not open the hand, hence the hand was of limited functional use. (Compare with Souques' phenomenon, discussed at the end of this chapter.)

INVESTIGATION OF ASSOCIATED REACTIONS BY SIMONS

An extensive investigation of associated reactions was undertaken by Simons, a German physician who became interested in these phenomena during World War I. At first, his observations were limited to patients who had suffered head injuries, but after the war he included other types of patients with hemiplegia in his studies (Simons, 1923).

Simons noticed that the position of the patient's head had a marked influence on the outcome of the associated limb reactions, and that these limb reactions closely resembled the tonic neck reflexes in decerebrate animals, which had been discovered a few years earlier by Magnus and de Kleijn. In decerebrate animals, passive head motions or stationary head positions had been found to evoke specific responses in the limbs. In human patients, however, Simons could observe little or no reflex effect from passive head movements. But a forceful muscular contraction on the normal side together with head positioning brought out limb movements which followed the rules formulated by Magnus and de Kleijn. Simons concluded that the reactions he observed in patients with hemiplegia were neck reflexes, but that reinforcements by muscular contractions in other parts of the body was required to evoke the reflexes. For reinforcement Simons routinely used forceful fist closure by having his patients squeeze an object in the normal hand.

STUDIES OF ASSOCIATED REACTIONS BY THE AUTHOR

Intrigued by Simons' observations and reports, the author eagerly studied associated reactions of patients with hemiplegia in the clinic for several years. It was hoped that some new training ideas would evolve from the study of the motor behavior of these patients. Such ideas were badly needed because, in the experience of the author, patients with hemiparesis did not respond very well to "muscle reeducation" as employed by physical therapists in the training of patients with lower motor neuron lesions.

A preliminary investigation of associated reactions was undertaken at the Kessler Institute for Rehabilitation, West Orange, N.J., during 1951 and 1952. Patients were tested in supine, prone, side-lying, sitting, and standing positions. The results observed usually confirmed Simons' findings that the position of the head in a predictable manner influenced the form of the associated reactions. This at least seemed to be the case when the reactions were evoked by having the patient firmly grip an object in the hand on the normal side, as recommended by Simons. But when resistance to a variety of limb movements was employed to evoke the responses, contradictory reactions, difficult to explain, often appeared.

It seemed of considerable interest, both from a theoretical and a practical standpoint, to determine if a definite relationship existed between the type of resisted movement employed and the ensuing associated reaction. A second study was therefore undertaken, this time at the Burke Rehabilitation Center, White Plains, N.Y., between March 1954 and May 1955 (Brunnstrom, 1956). At this time, training techniques began to evolve.

Because associated reactions had been found to be either flexion or extension in nature, the author wished to find out whether resistance to a flexor movement (or an extensor movement) on the normal side tended to evoke the *same* or the *opposite* type of movement on the affected side. Fist closure, as mostly used by Simons, was unsuitable for this purpose because the author had observed that finger flexion frequently accompanied both flexor and extensor responses.

The patients were examined in the supine position, first with the head in a neutral position, then with the head rotated left, then right, as resistance was given on the normal side. For each head position, the effect of type of resistance given was recorded.

The results of the investigation may be summarized as follows:

1. In the *upper limb* the reactions were of the same type as the movements employed to evoke the responses, i.e., *flexion tended to evoke flexion* and *extension tended to evoke extension.*
2. In the lower limb the reactions were of the opposite type to the movement

employed to evoke the responses, i.e., *flexion tended to evoke extension* and *extension tended to evoke flexion.*

The data also confirmed observations previously made, namely, that flexion predominates in the upper, extension in the lower limb.

A definite influence from the tonic neck reflexes on the associated responses was observed, but other influences were present as well. The outcome of the associated reactions apparently was determined by the summation of various sensorimotor influences, some of which were positive, others negative, with respect to flexion and extension.

ASSOCIATED REACTIONS EVOKED BY YAWNING, SNEEZING, AND COUGHING

A yawn in a patient with hemiplegia is frequently accompanied by involuntary muscular contractions in the affected upper limb. Usually, a flexor synergy develops during the inhalation phase of the yawn, and the reaction begins to fade out when the patient exhales. Some patients with hemiplegia state that when they yawn in the morning the affected arm reaches forward and the hand opens up. The latter reaction, however, is evoked not from a regular yawn but from a "morning stretch." Both types of reactions develop slowly, are of some duration, and disappear slowly. The stimulus must have an automatic character, because if the patient voluntarily initiates a yawn or a "morning stretch" the reactions do not develop.

Coughing and sneezing evoke sudden muscular contractions of short duration.

THE NATURE OF ASSOCIATED REACTIONS

Walshe, an English neurologist, points out that postural adjustments which are constantly needed during purposive movements are carried out by reflex mechanisms and that these mechanisms are operating in patients with hemiplegia, although the reflexes no longer adapt to the individual's needs. According to Walshe, "associated reactions are released postural reactions deprived of voluntary control" (Walshe, 1923b).

In the cases studied by Walshe, the latency of the associated reactions varied from 0.25 to 2.0 seconds. Phasic reflexes such as tendon jerks, Walshe points out, are characterized by short latency periods. As an example, in one of Walshe's patients the supinator jerk had a latency of 0.04 second, while in the same patient the associated reaction had a latency period of 0.74 second. Walshe concludes that "in respect to stimulus, latency, form and duration, the associated reaction presents all the characteristics of a tonic or postural reflex." (In animals, Magnus and de Kleijn [1912] found that the latency period for the tonic labyrinthine reflex varied between ⅓ and 23 seconds; for the tonic neck reflex the latency period varied between ⅓ and 6 seconds.)

HOMOLATERAL LIMB SYNKINESIS

A mutual dependency appears to exist between the synergies of the affected upper and lower limbs in patients with spastic hemiplegia. Thus, flexion of one of the limbs tends to evoke or facilitate a flexion of the other. Homolateral synkinesis manifests itself most clearly during reflexly evoked movements. The stimuli that elicit the responses may originate on the affected or on the unaffected side. Figures 1-13 and 1-14 are examples of homolateral synkinesis.

In Figure 1-13, resistance to elbow flexion on the affected side evokes flexion of the homolateral lower limb. The reaction appeared when the patient's head was in a neutral position (Fig. 1-13A), and it became reinforced from impulses originating in the neck when the head was rotated toward the normal side (Fig. 1-13B).

In Figure 1-14, homolateral synkinesis is evoked by unresisted inward rotation of the hip on the normal side. The reaction has the opposite character from the movement causing its appearance. (Inward rotation of the hip belongs to the extensor synergy; the response is flexor in nature.)

The theories of Fay concerning the motor behavior of children with cerebral palsy are of interest if one considers the significance of homolateral synkinesis in adult patients with hemiplegia. Fay points out that the homolateral pattern originated on the amphibian level of evolution, and that the crossed pattern represents a later (quadrupedal) motor performance. Fay observed that in children with cerebral palsy the crossed pattern develops from the homolateral pattern when the central nervous system of the child has reached the proper development (Fay, 1946, 1955).

Homolateral synkinesis in adult patients with hemiplegia would suggest that the nervous system, having reached its full development in these patients, has undergone "evolution in reverse" (Jackson, 1884) and that this reversal goes back to the amphibian level of evolution.

RAIMISTE'S PHENOMENA

A number of associated reactions characteristic of patients with hemiplegia that are different from those described in the previous pages were reported by Raimiste, a French neurologist.

The associated movements of abduction and adduction were discovered when Raimiste examined his patients for the purpose of comparing the muscular strength of the affected lower limb with that of the normal limb (Raimiste, 1909). Additional associated movements are discussed in a later report (1911).

The Abduction Phenomenon

In the supine position, arms crossed over the chest and the two limbs close together, the patient is asked to bring the normal limb out to the side without raising it off the bed. The examiner stands on the patient's normal side and opposes the movement by resisting on the lateral side of the limb. If the resistance is strong, the normal limb is held in place and the affected limb is seen to move into abduction (Fig. 1-15A).

The Adduction Phenomenon

In the supine position, with the arms crossed over the chest and the two legs spread apart, the patient is asked to bring his unaffected limb toward the affected one. This movement is firmly opposed by the examiner who resists on the medial side of the limb. When the patient attempts to carry out the requested movement an associated adduction of the affected limb occurs (Fig. 1-15B).

Raimiste points out that a tendency to move both legs simultaneously is present also in normal persons. If adduction is resisted on one side, a slight internal rotation of the hip on the opposite side may

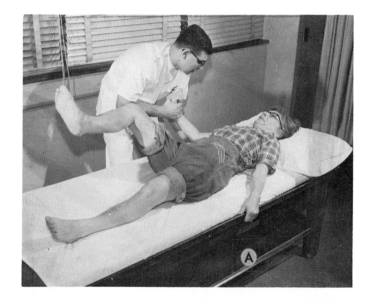

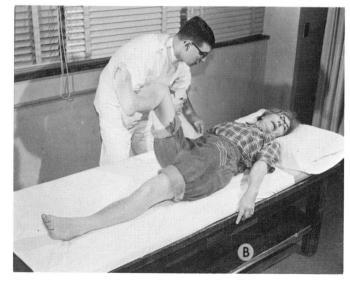

FIGURE 1-13. Associated flexor synergy of right lower limb, evoked by resistance to elbow flexion on the same side. The patient, age 48, had suffered a cerebral vascular accident 10 months earlier. *A.* With the head in a neutral position, a typical flexor synergy of the affected lower limb develops. *B.* Head rotation toward the normal side reinforces the associated reaction. (*A* from Brunnstrom, S. Motor testing procedures in hemiplegia. *J. Amer. Phys. Ther. Ass.* 46:357, 1966.)

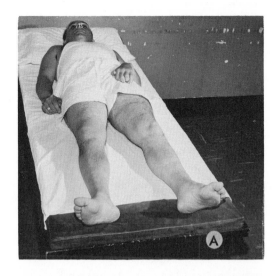

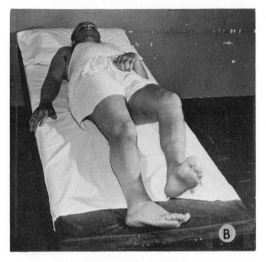

FIGURE 1-14. The patient, age 48, has a left-sided spastic hemiplegia of 5 months' standing. *A.* In the starting position patient is relaxed, but flexor tension in the upper limb remains. *B.* Forceful-inward rotation of the right hip evokes flexor responses in left upper and lower limbs. A homolateral pattern has developed on the affected side.

be noticed in normal persons, but adduction of the limb is seldom observed. If the normal person is told not to move the limb, he can easily control it. But the patient with hemiplegia cannot always prevent the movement and he frequently declares that the limb moved "all by itself."

The associated abduction and adduction movements are considered by Raimiste to be a sign of "organic" hemiplegia, as opposed to "hysteric" hemiplegia. Positive signs were observed in patients with recent as well as long-standing hemiplegia. Raimiste observed that the signs sometimes appeared earlier, sometimes later, than the Babinski sign.

In the experience of the author Raimiste's sign is positive in the largest number of patients with hemiplegia, regardless of whether or not voluntary control of abduction and adduction is present. Adduction is more easily evoked than abduction and is accompanied by internal rotation of the hip if resistance on the normal side is sustained. In some patients, several trials may be required before the phenomena appear.

The observation that adduction appears quite readily as compared to abduction may be explained as resulting from the influence of the extensor synergy. Because the hip and knee are already extended, adduction and internal rotation, which are extensor components, are facilitated and therefore ready to respond.

If the firm linkage between the synergy components were the only influence present, one would expect that abduction would be inhibited in the affected limb because abduction belongs to the flexor synergy. To a certain extent, this is true since abduction is found to be more difficult to elicit as an associated reaction than adduction. But another force must be present which has stronger influence than the synergies, or no abduction would materialize.

The probable nature of the abduction and adduction signs was discussed by Raimiste and also by other French neurologists. The opinion was expressed that the signs are related to a facilitating effect that is inherent in symmetrical movements. This effect is present under normal circumstances, and it is exaggerated in hemiplegia. Marie and Foix (1916) admit that this may be the case, but prefer to classify the abduction and adduction phenomena as "coordination synkinesis."

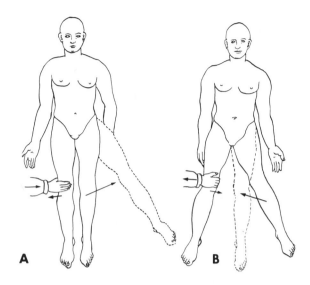

FIGURE 1-15. Raimiste's phenomena. (Redrawn from Marie and Foix, 1916.) *A.* The patient is asked to abduct the normal limb while the therapist opposes the movement. Result: associated abduction of the affected limb. *B.* The patient is asked to adduct the normal limb while the therapist opposes the movement. Result: associated adduction of the affected limb.

It has previously been stated that in the lower limb the associated response is generally of the opposite type from the stimulus by means of which it is evoked; that is, flexion evokes extension, and extension evokes flexion. In Raimiste's phenomenon, on the other hand, the stimulus and the response are of the same type—that is, abduction evokes abduction, and adduction evokes adduction. This may seem confusing at first, but the symmetry of the movements may explain the matter.

A reaction akin to Raimiste's adduction phenomenon, observed by the author in the upper extremity of patients with hemiplegia, concerns a bilateral response of the pectoralis major muscle. The reaction, as employed for training purposes, is described in Chapter 3.

HAND REACTIONS

The evolution of the grasping function of the human hand may be traced back to the simple stretch reflex, a spinal cord reaction. In successive steps, as a result of activities on higher levels of the central nervous system, this reaction is transformed into more and more elaborate mechanisms until adult human hand function has evolved (Denny-Brown, 1956; Twitchell, 1958).

Restoration of hand function following hemiplegia in man proceeds in a manner that closely resembles the evolutionary one. From data collected during a clinical study, Twitchell (1951) outlined seven steps in the restoration of function of these patients, as follows:

1. Tendon reflexes return and become hyperactive.
2. Spasticity develops; resistance to passive motions is felt.
3. Voluntary finger flexion occurs, if facilitated by proprioceptive stimuli.
4. The "proprioceptive traction response" (see below) can be elicited.
5. Control of hand movements without proprioceptive stimuli begins.
6. Grasp is greatly reinforced by tactile stimuli in the palm of the hand. Spasticity is declining.
7. The true grasp reflex (see below) can be elicited. Spasticity has decreased further.

In the majority of the patients studied by Twitchell, recovery ceased before the last stage had been reached; it could be arrested anywhere along the line. A small group of patients—those who exhibited the grasp reflex—progressed to full recovery, that is, movements could be performed with speed and skill equal to that of the uninvolved side. At the time when the grasp reflex appeared, extension of the fingers was greatly improved; prior to this time, finger extension had been slow and awkward.

THE PROPRIOCEPTIVE TRACTION RESPONSE

This response, also referred to as the proximal traction response, has the following characteristics: a stretch of the flexor muscles of one of the joints of the upper limb—any joint—evokes or facilitates contraction of the flexor muscles of all the other joints so that a total shortening of the limb may result. Twitchell observed that the traction response was markedly facilitated or inhibited by the tonic neck reflex in accordance with the rules formulated by Magnus and de Kleijn.

Twitchell also observed an influence of the body-righting reflexes on the traction response in the patients studied. When the patient was lying on his side with the affected limbs on the upper side, the traction response was facilitated; when lying on the affected side, the response was inhibited. This finding was interpreted as a manifestation of the body-righting reflex. The reflex status of these patients corresponds to the reflex posture of thalamic monkeys described by Magnus (1922) and referred to by Bieber and Fulton (1938). The distribution of tone in the extremities in these animals is expressed as "flexion of the uppermost, extension of the underlying extremities."

THE TRUE GRASP REFLEX

The true grasp reflex was described by Seyffarth and Denny-Brown (1948). It is elicited by a distally moving deep pressure over certain areas of the palmar surface of hand and digits as indicated in Figure 1-16. It is imperative that the stimulus move in a distal direction, because a proximally moving stimulus has no effect. The reflexo-

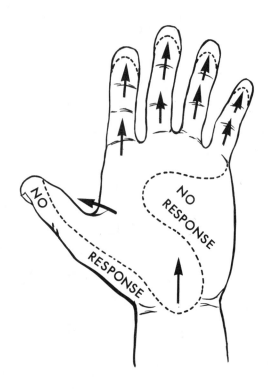

FIGURE 1-16. Diagram showing the regions of the palmar side of the hand from which the grasp reflex can be elicited (see text). (Redrawn from Seyffarth and Denny-Brown, 1948.)

genic zone begins on the palmar surface of the wrist and includes most of the palm (except the ulnar portion). Response is obtained over metacarpophalangeal and interphalangeal joints of all five digits; it is weakest over the thumb joints. The response from these local areas consists of flexion of the joint or joints over which the stimulus moves. A positive response from any local area momentarily reinforces the reaction in other local areas. Stimulation in between any two digits in a palmar-dorsal direction evokes adduction of the neighboring digits.

The grasp reflex has two phases, a *catching phase* and a *holding phase*. The catching phase consists of weak contractions of flexor and adductor muscles. The holding phase appears only if traction is made on the tendons of the muscles activated during the catching phase; it continues as long as the traction on the muscles is sustained.

Denny-Brown (1956) discusses the relationship between the proprioceptive traction response and the grasp reflex. The traction response is elicited by stretch—that is, proprioceptors are involved—while the grasp reflex is evoked by a tactile stimulus. Once this tactile stimulus has produced a response (catching phase), stretch of muscles causes the traction response to appear (holding phase). Because the traction response is absent prior to the catching phase, it is the contactual stimulus that has "triggered" the proprioceptive response.

THE INSTINCTIVE GRASP REACTION

The term *instinctive grasp reaction* is suggested by Seyffarth and Denny-Brown (1948) to distinguish it from the grasp reflex. The lack of uniformity of terms used by previous investigators, such as "grasp reflex," "closure reflex," "the palmar reflex," "forced grasping," "forced groping," "tonic perserveration," and "tonic innervation," also impelled the authors to reexamine and define these phenomena.

The adequate stimulus for the instinctive grasp reaction is a *stationary contact* with the palm of the hand, while the grasp reflex requires a moving stimulus. A person who exhibits the instinctive grasp reaction is compelled to close the hand over an object that comes in contact with the palm of the hand (Fig. 1-17). Once involuntary fist closure has been completed, the person is unable to release the object. Without an object in the hand, however, he has no difficulty in opening and closing the hand. If an object comes in contact with portions of the hand other than the palm, small orienting movements by the hand occur until the palmar side of the hand is close to the object. Such preliminary movements constitute "forced groping" described by other authors.

The instinctive grasp reaction is present at birth, but subsequently disappears. Because the reaction may appear in adult persons with brain damage, Denny-Brown concludes that it has been suppressed during the maturation process of the nervous system, but it has not been lost.

The person in Figure 1-17 displayed a typical instinctive grasp reaction. The involvement of the left upper limb was mild; the arm could be moved voluntarily in all directions, and no synergy influence was detected. When the hand was empty, the person opened and closed the hand freely. But if a small object, such as a ball or a pencil or the examiner's two fingers, were placed in her palm, the fist automatically closed around the object. When the examiner attempted to withdraw her fingers the grip tightened. Even though she concentrated on the task, the patient was unable to prevent a fist closure or to release the grip after it had developed. However, fist closure could be prevented if the examiner quickly stimulated the

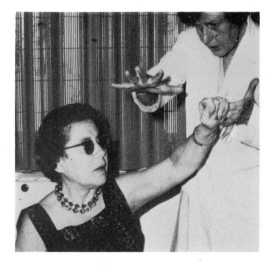

FIGURE 1-17. The instinctive grasp reaction. Fist closes automatically over object touching the palm of the hand. Patient is unable to release the grasp. Condition has been unchanged for 14 years following surgery for a brain abscess. (Frame of a motion picture.)

dorsum of the hand as closure began; a fraction of a second later such stimulation was ineffective. The only way that the patient could release the object was to palmar flex the wrist with her other hand while the affected hand rested in the lap and the entire arm was relaxed.

A second patient, age 60, who exhibited the instinctive grasp reaction was seen by the author. As in the preceding case, the patient could open and close the empty hand without difficulty, but contact of an object with the palm of the hand resulted in a rapid involuntary fist closure. "It is like a trap," the patient commented. "I can't help it." When the patient opposed his thumb to one finger after the other, a clonic tremor of flexion-extension of the metacarpophalangeal joints developed, a symptom not observed in the first case.

Sequences in the Restoration of Grasp. Neurophysiologically, restoration of the grasping function of the hand in patients with hemiplegia, as outlined by Denny-Brown and Twitchell, has the following sequence.

Recovery begins with the return of the stretch reflex, a monosegmental spinal cord reflex. It is followed by the proprioceptive traction response, a plurisegmental response involving centers higher than the spinal cord. Next comes the grasp reflex, a subcortical response. From it evolves the instinctive grasp reaction, which is said to have a cortical component. Finally, by inhibition of the instinctive grasp reaction, complete control of grasp and release is established.

THE INSTINCTIVE AVOIDING REACTION

The instinctive grasp reaction may be observed in patients with lesions of the frontal lobe; the instinctive avoiding reaction occurs in patients with parietal lobe lesions (Denny-Brown, 1956).

The avoiding reaction is illustrated in Figure 1-18. When the arm of this patient was held elevated in a forward-upward direction, the fingers, including the thumb, hyperextended in a characteristic fashion. Stroking over the palmar surface of the hand in a distal direction caused an exaggeration of the hand posture (Fig. 1-18A). The stroking was delivered in the center of the palm of the hand, and the fingers responded before the stimulus had reached the metacarpophalangeal joint of the middle finger.

When the patient reached out to grasp an object, the fingers again overextended (Fig. 1-18B). The grasping of the object could be completed but was preceded by a momentary hesitation, as though a special concentration were required to make the hand obey.

The person whose hand is shown in Figure 1-18 had good control of free flexion and extension of the fingers and used the hand for many activities, although with a slight awkwardness. The disability was said to have developed following an automobile accident that had occurred nine years earlier. Her history indicated that she had been an inmate in a psychiatric hospital, but whether her psychotic condition had any relation to the appearance of the avoiding reaction is not known. (Compare with discussion by Denny-Brown, 1956.)

The overextension phenomenon is relatively common in children with cerebral palsy (Twitchell, 1958). It was observed that in such children a stimulation on the ulnar side of the palm was the most effective, and that some children responded only in this region; in other children responses were obtained from all areas of the palm. The weakness of grasp seen in these children, Twitchell suggests, may well be related to the avoiding reaction, because an object in the hand may evoke a reaction that is antagonistic to the child's voluntary grasping effort.

Throughout the nervous system there exists a "competition" between antagonistic reflex impulses. Normally, neuromuscular

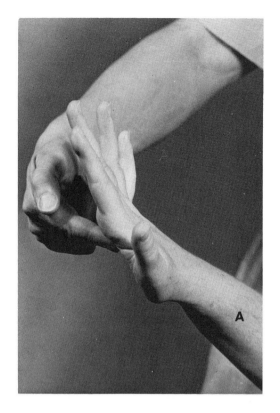

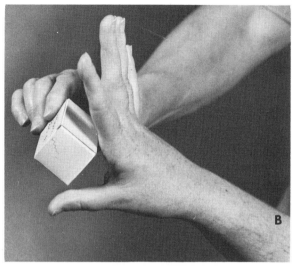

FIGURE 1-18. The instinctive avoiding reaction. Patient, age 43, appeared to move her right arm in a normal fashion, but displayed the overextension phenomenon described by Denny-Brown (1956) and by Twitchell (1958). *A.* The patient's right arm is held elevated by the examiner who stimulates the palmar surface of the hand. An exaggerated extension of all digits is evoked. *B.* The patient reaches out to grasp an object. As the affected hand approaches the object, the fingers hyperextend.

impulses of opposite character keep each other in balance, but in the presence of pathology such balance may be disturbed. If the source of one set of impulses is affected by pathology and the antagonistic set is intact, impaired motor function may result because of overactivity of the intact mechanism. On the cortical level, the instinctive grasp reaction and the instinctive avoiding reaction constitute an antagonistic pair (Denny-Brown, 1956). When the source of the instinctive avoiding reaction (located in the frontal lobe) is affected by disease or injury, the instinctive grasp reaction is released, a phenomenon described by Denny-Brown as "transcortical release." Conversely, pathology at the source of the instinctive grasp reaction (located in the parietal lobe) results in release of the instinctive avoiding reaction. These conclusions were drawn from ablation experiments on monkeys.

SOUQUES' FINGER PHENOMENON

This phenomenon is referred to in the French literature and discussed by Marie and Foix (1916). Souques observed that in patients with hemiplegia an elevation of the affected arm frequently caused the paralyzed fingers to extend automatically, but he states that the reaction is not observable in all patients with hemiplegia.

The author has observed Souques' phenomenon in a considerable number of

31

patients with hemiplegia. The patient in Figure 1-14 had marked spasticity in the flexor muscles of wrist and fingers; yet, when the arm was passively raised overhead the fist opened and the fingers extended in a queer fashion. A second patient with mild involvement of the right arm as a result of a head injury was able to close the hand in all arm postures but could open the hand only in the overhead position. If the arm was passively lowered by small increments, finger extension became more and more difficult and the range of extension diminished rapidly. Fist opening became impossible by the time the arm was half way down. A third patient who had voluntary control of fist closure and fist opening in all arm postures had a reaction that might also be interpreted as a manifestation of the same phenomenon. Whenever the arm was raised by the examiner the fingers extended fully, appearing to do so automatically, regardless of their previous position. This reaction was observed repeatedly when the patient's attention was focused elsewhere; he appeared to be unaware of the opening of the hand.

To judge from the three cases cited above, of which one patient was severely involved, the other two much less affected, it would seem that the finger extension phenomenon observed by Souques does not characterize any particular recovery stage. Numerous clinical observations by the author suggests that, to some extent, finger extension is facilitated in the overhead position of the arm in all patients with hemiplegia, even though automatic finger extension materializes in only relatively few cases. For training purposes, the elevated arm position has proved favorable in many patients (see Chapter 3).

REFERENCES

Beevor, C. E. *The Croonian Lectures on Muscular Movement,* delivered in 1903. Edited and reprinted for the Guarantors of *Brain.* New York, Macmillan, 1951, pp. 44–47.

Bieber, I., and Fulton, J. F. Relation of the cerebral cortex to the grasp reflex and the postural and righting reflexes. *Arch. Neurol. Psychiat.* 39:433, 1938.

Bobath, K., and Bobath, B. O. Treatment of cerebral palsy by the inhibition of abnormal reflex action. *Brit. Orthopt. J.* 11:88, 1954.

Brunnstrom, S. Associated reactions of the upper extremity in adult patients with hemiplegia. *Phys. Ther. Rev.* 36:225, 1956.

Byers, R. K. Tonic neck reflexes in children. Considered from a diagnostic standpoint. *Amer. J. Dis. Child.* 55:696, 1938.

Denny-Brown, D. Positive and negative aspects of cerebral cortical functions. *N. Carolina Med. J.* 17:295, 1956.

Doman, R. J., Spitz, E. B., Zucman, E., Delacato, C. H., and Doman, G. Children with severe brain injuries. *J. Amer. Med. Ass.* 174:257, 1960.

Fay, T. Observation on the rehabilitation of movement in cerebral palsy problems. *W. Virginia Med J.* 42:77, 1946.

Fay, T. The origin of human movement. *Amer. J. Psychiat.* 111:644, 1955.

Gesell, A., Halverson, H. M., Ilg, F. L., Thompson, H. Castner, B. M., Ames, L. B., and Amatruda, C. S. *The First Five Years of Life. The Preschool Years.* New York, Harper & Row, 1940, Part I.

Gesell, A., and Ames, L. B. Tonic neck reflexes and symmetro-tonic behavior. *J. Pediat.* 36:165, 1950.

Hellebrandt, F. A., Houtz, S. J. Partridge, M. J., and Walters, C. E. Tonic neck reflexes in exercises of stress in man. *Amer. J. Phys. Med.* 35:144, 1956.

Hoff, H. E. Labyrinthine and neck reflexes in single motor neurones of soleus muscle. *Amer. J. Physiol.* 105:54, 1933.

Ikay, M. Tonic neck reflexes in normal persons. *Jap. J. Physiol.* 1:118, 1950.

Jackson, J. H. "Evolution and Dissolution of the Nervous System" (1884), in *Selected Writings of John Hughlings Jackson,* ed. by J. Taylor. New York, Basic Books, 1958, p. 45–75.

Magnus, R., and de Kleijn, A. Die Abhängigkeit des Tonus der Extremitätenmuskeln von der Kopfstellung. *Pflüger Arch. Physiol.* 145:455, 1912.

Marie, P., and Foix, C. Les syncinésies des hémiplégiques. *Rev. Neurol.* 29:3, 1916, and 30:146, 1916.

Raimiste, J. Deux signes d'hémiplégie organique du membre inférieur. *Rev. Neurol.* 17:125, 1909.

RAIMISTE, J. Sur les mouvements associés du membre inférieur malade chez les hémiplégiques organiques. *Rev. Neurol.* 21:71, 1911.

RIDDOCH, G., and BUZZARD, E. F. Reflex movements and postural reactions in quadriplegia and hemiplegia, with special reference to those of the upper limb. *Brain* 44:397, 1921.

SCHALTENBRANDT, G. The development of human motility and motor disturbances. *Arch. Neurol. Psychiat.* 20:720, 1928.

SEYFFARTH, H., and DENNY-BROWN, D. The grasp reflex and the instinctive grasp reaction. *Brain* 71:109, 1948.

SIMONS, A. Kopfhaltung und Muskeltonus, klinische Beobachtungen. *Z. Neurol.* 80:499, 1923.

TOKIZANE, T., MURAO, M., OGATA, T., and KENDO, T. Electromyographic studies on tonic neck, lumbar and labyrinthine reflexes in normal persons. *Jap. J. Physiol.* 2:130, 1951.

TWITCHELL, T. E. The restoration of motor function following hemiplegia in man. *Brain* 74:443, 1951.

TWITCHELL, T. E. The grasping deficit in infantile spastic hemiparesis. *Neurology* 8:13, 1958.

WALSHE, F. M. R. A case of complete decerebrate rigidity in man. *Lancet* 205:644, 1923a.

WALSHE, F. M. R. On certain tonic or postural reflexes in hemiplegia with special reference to the so-called "associated movements." *Brain* 46:1, 1923b.

WATERLAND, C., and HELLEBRANDT, F. A. Involuntary patterning associated with willed movement performed against progressively increasing resistance. *Amer. J. Phys. Med.* 34:13, 1964.

2

Recovery
Stages and
Evaluation
Procedures

RECOVERY STAGES:
BASIS FOR EVALUATION

In observing a large number of patients with hemiplegia for longer or shorter periods of time, the author has been impressed by the almost stereotyped sequences of events that take place during recovery. Immediately following the acute episode, flaccidity is present and no movements of the limbs can be initiated (Stage 1). As recovery begins, the basic limb synergies or some of their components may appear as associated reactions, or minimal voluntary movement responses may be present. At this time spasticity begins to develop (Stage 2). Thereafter, the patient gains voluntary control of the movement synergies, although full range of all synergy components does not necessarily develop. Spasticity has further increased and may become severe (Stage 3). Then some movement combinations that do not follow the paths of either synergy are mastered, first with difficulty, then with more ease, and spasticity begins to decline (Stage 4). If progress continues, more difficult movement combinations are learned as the basic limb synergies lose their dominance over motor acts (Stage 5). With the disappearance of spasticity, individual joint movements become possible and coordination approaches normal (Stage 6). From here on, as the last recovery step, normal motor function is restored, but this last stage is not included on the evaluation form.

The above recovery sequences were established empirically from clinical observations of 26 patients at the Burke Rehabilitation Center during 1954 and 1955, and 74 patients at the Institute of Rehabilitation Medicine, New York City, between 1955 and 1956. The validity of these observations has been subsequently confirmed over the years.

DEVELOPMENT OF THE EVALUATION FORM

Considerable time was required for the development of an adequate evaluation form. Several types of forms were tried and found unsatisfactory. Originally, a large number of movement combinations and functional activities were tested. As more experience was gained, test items that appeared to duplicate one another were eliminated until only a few movement combinations, representative of a particular recovery stage, were retained. The principle that a clinical evaluation of this kind must be brief, yet clearly indicate sequences of progress, was adhered to throughout the elimination process.

In an effort to measure progress in every detail, one is tempted to add more and more test items, but then the procedure becomes too time consuming. Should specific additions be indicated for individual patients, it is better to write an explanatory note than to burden the form with items that are not essential for most patients.

The first evaluation form for the upper limb that closely resembles the one presently used was published by Reynolds and associates (1958). This form was originally developed for a clinical research project to seek information, among other things, about the effect of afferent stimuli on the patient's motor performance. The form was found to be too long for ordinary clinical use and had to be revised. The revised form, presented here, requires less time, partly because the recording of the effects of afferent stimuli has been eliminated, partly because a number of items have been omitted. The form can be further abbreviated if less sensory information and fewer details of motor performance are required.

PRINCIPLES FOR EVALUATING PROGRESS IN HEMIPLEGIA

A test to evaluate neuromuscular progress of patients with hemiplegia must, at least to a certain extent, reflect the condition of those portions of the central nervous system that regulate motor performance. By having the patients perform, or attempt to perform, selected motor acts requiring increasingly finer neuromuscular control, an assessment of the degree of recovery of the central nervous system can be made. This approach differs from the approach used in evaluating muscular strength alone.

To be acceptable, the procedure employed to evaluate progress of patients with hemiplegia should:

1. Be based on the typical recovery stages of these patients, as an indication of the approximate extent of the recovery of the central nervous system
2. Be brief and easy to administer so as not to fatigue the patient too much and not to encroach unduly on the time available for training purposes
3. Avoid complicated equipment, yet the procedure should function with a considerable amount of objectivity
4. Be standardized and administered by personnel familiar with the motor behavior of patients with hemiplegia

The well-known manual "muscle test," which was originally devised by Dr. R. W. Lovett in Boston for testing progress of postpoliomyelitis patients (Lovett, 1917), does not meet the criteria outlined above. In testing patients with lower motor neuron lesions, *individual joint movements* are employed. The testing criterion is *strength,* as measured by the subject's ability to perform movements of body segments with gravity eliminated, against gravity, and against gravity and added resistance.

In hemiplegia, individual joint movements cannot be performed as long as spasticity is present; therefore, movement patterns, not individual joint movements, must be tested. Furthermore, the tension which a muscle group can produce varies a great deal according to numerous cir-

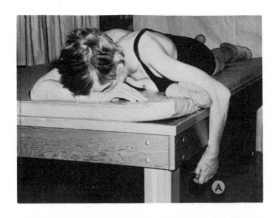

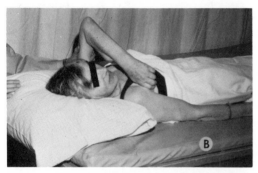

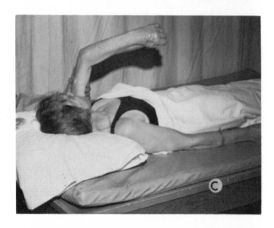

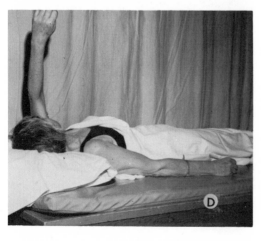

cumstances, such as the position of the patient (supine, prone, side-lying, sitting, standing), the position of the head in relation to the trunk, the position of limb segments with respect to each other, and simultaneous activities in associated muscle groups. Strength, per se, therefore, cannot be used as a criterion.

Figure 2-1 illustrates the effect of the prone and the supine positions on elbow extension in a patient with hemiplegia. In the prone position, even with greatest effort, the patient was unable to extend the elbow (Fig. 2-1A), but in the supine position, the elbow was extended full range (Fig. 2-1B–D). The patient might even have been able to extend against gravity and added resistance, because resistance reinforces the muscular contraction. If one were to use the conventional "muscle test," in the supine position the elbow extensor muscles would be graded Fair or Better, while this grade would not apply to the prone position. When sitting with the arm supported on a horizontal smooth surface, a patient with spastic hemiplegia would be unable to extend the elbow in a side-horizontal direction, but elbow extension in a forward-horizontal direction might succeed full range. (In the latter direction, all components of the extensor synergy are allowed to participate; in the former direction, the pectoralis major muscle must be inhibited.) Should the elbow extensor muscles of such a patient be graded Less than Poor, Fair, Fair Plus, or perhaps Good? The physical therapist who is expected to give a "muscle test" to a patient with spastic hemiplegia certainly has a problem on his hands!

FIGURE 2-1. Influence of the prone and supine positions on elbow extension in 71-year-old woman with left-sided hemiparesis, 3 months after cerebral vascular accident. *A.* The patient makes an effort to extend the elbow but the elbow *flexes* tightly over the edge of the table. *B, C,* and *D.* In the supine position, the patient extends the elbow full range. Light stabilization of the arm is required.

Similar difficulties are encountered if one attempts to test muscles in the lower extremity. For example, it may be impossible for the patient to use the quadriceps muscles to perform isolated knee extension in the side-lying position (gravity eliminated); yet, the quadriceps muscles may contract vigorously when, in standing, the patient shifts his weight to the affected limb. Another example is the behavior of the muscles that dorsiflex the ankle. In the supine position, legs extended, the patient may be unable to initiate a contraction of these muscles. But when voluntary hip flexion is performed, the dorsiflexor muscles of the ankle may contract vigorously, and considerable resistance may be applied, not only to the hip, but also to the ankle movement.

THE VALIDITY OF THE EVALUATION PROCEDURE

To answer the question of whether the six stages on the evaluation form actually represent sequential recovery stages in a large number of patients, statistics were compiled on 118 patients in two groups. The first group of 65 patients (32 males and 33 females between 22 and 88 years) were examined at the Neurological Institute, New York City, during 1961 and 1962. The time which had elapsed from the onset of hemiplegia to the time the evaluation was given varied from 5 days to 5 years. The second group of patients (23 males and 30 females between 15 and 85 years) were evaluated during 1965 and 1966.

In going over the results of the tests, as well as a large number of progress notes, it became clear that every patient could be classified in one or another of the six recovery stages and that the evaluation form, as designed, conforms to the criteria of sequential recovery. In the 1961–1962 group, 33 out of 65 patients had been evaluated two to six times, the remaining 32 patients only once. In the 1965–1966 group

only a relatively small number had been reevaluated. The patients who were tested more than once either progressed in an orderly fashion from one stage to the next or made little or no progress and remained in the stage of the first evaluation; no patients skipped any of the stages.

A slight variation in performance was observed in Stages 4 and 5, inasmuch as an item chosen for Stage 5 was performed, or partially performed, before all three items listed in Stage 4 had been mastered. As a rule, however, the progression was exactly as indicated on the form.

Because progress is gradual, no absolute demarcation line can be established between the stages. In some instances, therefore, a 2–3, 3–4, 4–5, or 5–6 classification may be given to indicate that the patient is in the process of moving from one stage to the next.

RECORDING ACHIEVEMENT ON EVALUATION FORM

STANDARDIZATION OF TECHNIQUE

If this type of evaluation form is to become generally accepted by the medical and paramedical professions, a detailed standardization of technique would be required so that recordings at various institutions would have the same meaning. Such a standardization would best be accomplished by the joint effort of rehabilitation personnel from a number of hospitals and rehabilitation centers where the form here presented as Chart 1 (or a revision of the form) had been used long enough for the personnel to become familiar with its rationale and its administration.

For the time being, it is suggested that personnel at institutions wishing to experiment with this type of evaluation develop their own version of the form along with rules for its administration.

The discussion that follows provides only the most essential directions for the recording of status and progress of patients

Chart 1

HEMIPLEGIA—CLASSIFICATION AND PROGRESS RECORD (p. 1)
Upper Limb—Test Sitting

Name_____Age_____Date of onset_____Side affected_____

Date

_____ Passive motion sense, shoulder_____elbow_____

_____ pron.-supin._____wrist flex.-ext._____

_____ 1. NO MOVEMENT INITIATED OR ELICITED_____

_____ 2. SYNERGIES OR COMPONENTS FIRST APPEARING. Spasticity developing_____

_____   Flexor synergy_____

_____   Extensor synergy_____

_____ 3. SYNERGIES OR COMPONENTS INITIATED VOLUNTARILY. Spasticity marked_____

	FLEXOR SYNERGY	Active Joint Range		Remarks
	Shoulder girdle	Elevation			
		Retraction			
	Shoulder joint	Hyperextension Abduction			
		Ext. rotation			
	Elbow	Flexion			
	Forearm	Supination			
	EXTENSOR SYNERGY				
	Shoulder	Pectoralis major			
	Elbow	Extension			
	Forearm	Pronation			
	4. MOVEMENTS DEVIATING FROM BASIC SYNERGIES Spasticity decreasing	Hand to sacral region			
		Raise arm forw.-horiz.			
		Pron.-supin. elbow at 90°			
	5. RELATIVE IN-DEPENDENCE OF BASIC SYNERGIES Spasticity waning	Raise arm side-horiz.			
		Raise arm over head			
		Pron.-supin. elbow extended			
	6. MOVEMENT COORDINATION NEAR NORMAL. Spasticity minimal				

Chart 1 (Continued)

Upper Limb—Test Sitting (continued)

Name_____

Date

_____ SPEED TESTS for classes 4, 5, 6   Strokes per 5 sec.

Hand from lap to chin	Normal		
	Affected		
Hand from lap to opposite knee	Normal		
	Affected		

_____ Passive motion sense, digits_____

_____ Fingertip recognition_____

_____ Wrist stabilization 1. Elbow extended_____
             for grasp
                                2. Elbow flexed_____

_____ Wrist flexion   1. Elbow extended_____
             and extension
_____ fist closed   2. Elbow flexed_____

_____ Wrist circumduction_____

DIGITS

_____ Mass grasp_____Dynamometer test Normal_____lb.
                                                                      Affected_____lb.

_____ Mass extension_____

_____ Hook grasp (handbag, 2 lb.)_____

_____ Lateral prehension (card)_____

_____ Palmar prehension (pencil)_____

_____ Cylindrical grasp (small jar)_____

_____ Spherical grasp (ball)_____catch_____throw_____

_____ Indiv. thumb movements 1. Vertical movements_____
             hands in lap
_____ ulnar side down   2. Horizontal movements_____

_____ Individual finger movements_____

_____ Button and   Using both hands_____
             unbutton
_____ shirt   Using affected hand only_____

_____ Other skilled activities_____

Chart 1 (Continued)

HEMIPLEGIA—CLASSIFICATION AND PROGRESS RECORD (p. 3)
Trunk and Lower Limb

Name_____ Evaluation date_____

SUPINE

Passive   Hip_____Knee_____
motion
sense   Ankle_____Big toe_____

Flexor synergy_____

Extensor synergy_____

Hip: abduction_____adduction_____

SITTING ON CHAIR	STANDING
Trunk balance (no back support)	With_____Without_____support Balance, normal limb sec.
Sole sensation Correct (no. of answers) Incorrect	Double scale (a) (b) reading†
Hip-knee-ankle flexion	Hip-knee-ankle flexion
Knee flex.-ext. small range	Knee flex.-ext. small range
Knee flexion beyond 90°	Knee flexion Hip extended
Ankle, isolated dorsiflexion	Ankle, isolated dorsiflexion
Reciprocal hamstring action*	Hip abduction knee extended

AMBULATION   Evaluation date_____

Brace?_____Cane?_____In parallel bars_____

Supported_____Escorted_____Alone_____

Arm in sling_____Arm swings loosely_____Elbow held flexed_____

Arm swings near normal_____

GAIT ANALYSIS   Evaluation date _____

Stance Phase	Swing Phase
Ankle_____	_____
Knee_____	_____
Hip_____	_____

Walking cadence: Steps/min.   Speed: Feet/min.

*Inward and outward rotation at knee with inversion-eversion at ankle
†Recorded as normal/affected; (a) preferred stance; (b) weight shift on affected limb

with hemiplegia. The forms are designed primarily for testing motor achievement, but a brief investigation of the patient's sensory status has been included to serve as a guide for motor training. The sensory evaluation precedes motor evaluation.

GROSS TESTING FOR SENSORY LOSS

The significant aspects of sensation chosen for investigation are related to the patient's ability to recognize movements of the affected limbs, localization of touch in the hand, and appreciation of pressure in the sole of the foot. These tests purport to supply gross information only, information which will to a certain extent elucidate the patient's sensorimotor difficulties and aid in the planning of movement therapy. In no way is the sensory evaluation intended to take the place of a more accurate sensory examination carried out by other personnel.

Passive Motion Sense, Shoulder, Elbow, Forearm, and Wrist

As a preliminary procedure and to ascertain that the patient fully understands his role, the test is rehearsed as follows.

With the patient seated, the affected upper limb is supported by the investigator and moved to different positions while the patient observes the movement and performs identically with the unaffected limb (Fig. 2-2A). This rehearsal also gives the investigator an opportunity to gain the necessary skill in supporting the limb so that no change of grip is needed throughout the passive motion sequence. Simultaneously, it may be determined what movements, if any, are painful and in what muscle groups spasticity is present. A knowledge of the movement range in which resistance to passive movement is encountered is thus obtained in advance of the test.

Following rehearsal, the patient is blindfolded and the actual test is given. The affected limb is moved into new positions, involving shoulder, elbow, forearm, and wrist. Painful movements and the stretching of spastic muscles to the point where resistance is felt are avoided during testing. As before, the patient performs with his unaffected limb (Fig. 2-2B and C). The patient shown recognized shoulder and elbow movements fairly well, but neither wrist movements nor pronation-supination movements of the forearm were properly distinguished.

When a test of this kind is given to a blindfolded subject with normal sensation, he immediately indicates the change in joint position on one side by copying the movement on the other side. Patients with hemiplegia often hesitate before they respond because they are not sure that they are interpreting the sensation correctly. Some patients would rather make a guess than admit that they do not know the position of the limb. Wild guessing is easily discovered by additional test movements.

Passive Motion Sense, Digits (page 2 of evaluation form)

The patient is seated, with the pronated forearms resting on a firm pillow in his lap. The test is given with the patient blindfolded after a rehearsal without blindfold. The hands are relaxed and the fingers protrude over the edge of the pillow. One finger at a time is passively moved at the metacarpophalangeal joint in the direction of flexion or extension. If the patient feels the movement, he indicates its direction by saying "Up" or "Down." Aphasic patients may demonstrate the direction with the unaffected hand.

Fingertip Recognition (page 2 of evaluation form)

The patient's hands are positioned as in the preceding procedure, and the palmar surface of each of his fingertips is lightly touched with the rubber end of a pencil. The sequence of contact with the fingertips is irregular. The patient's task is to determine, without looking, which fingertip is being touched. Many patients fail to indicate the correct finger, and some do not distinguish a light touch at all.

Passive Motion Sense, Lower Limb (page 3 of evaluation form)

The lower limb is tested similarly to the upper limb. This test is conveniently administered with the patient in the supine position. The affected limb is carried by the examiner and supported in such a manner that movements can be performed without change of grip while testing hip, knee, and ankle. As the test begins, the patient's unaffected limb is flexed at hip and knee, and the sole of the foot is flat on the supporting surface. This position represents a midposition from which the patient can depart to indicate the change in position of the affected limb as the test is carried out.

Sole Sensation

In the lower limb an attempt is made to evaluate some aspects of sole sensation, mainly pressure, because such sensation is

important in order to recognize the quality of the walking surface. The test was originally given with the patient standing but was later given with the patient sitting. In sitting, balancing problems are all but eliminated, and the influence of various types of shoes—rubber or leather soles, thick or thin soles—can be avoided by having the patient remove his shoes. Both right and left sides are tested so that a comparison between the two sides can be made.

A narrow flat object, such as two tongue depressors taped together, is used in the test. It is shown to the patient. He is told that he has to determine, without looking, whether or not this object has been placed (1) under the foot, (2) all the way across the ball of the foot in a side-to-side direc-

FIGURE 2-2. Testing passive motion sense in 65-year-old patient with right-sided hemiparesis, 2½ months following removal of an intracranial abscess. (Frames of a motion picture.) *A.* Test is rehearsed (see text). *B.* For actual test, patient is blindfolded, he fails to recognize position of wrist. *C.* Position of forearm (supination) also is unrecognized. The patient's hesitance is reflected in his head position.

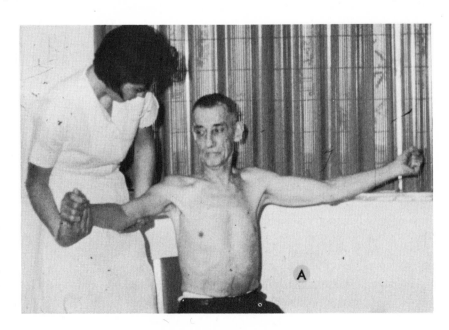

tion, (3) under only the medial side of the foot, or (4) under only the lateral side of the foot. The investigator exerts pressure downward on the foot to simulate weight bearing. The patient thus has four choices: (1) nothing under the foot, (2) object all the way across, (3) object on the side of the little toe, (4) object under the side of the great toe. Because the angles of the ankle joints change when an object is placed under the ball of the foot or under one side of the foot, and because of the necessity of handling the limb, this test involves several categories of sensations.

MOTOR TESTS: SHOULDER AND ELBOW

The patient is seated, preferably in a chair without arm rests. Before the test begins, it must be ascertained whether or not he can sit erect without side supports. If not, he may use a wheelchair or remain in bed. Beginning with Stage 3, testing is routinely done with the patient seated.

Recovery Stage 1 (Initial Stage)

A patient is classified in Stage 1 when no voluntary movement of the affected limb can be initiated. This classification is

frequently made while the patient is still confined to bed. Trunk movements may then be fairly well under control, but the patient is often too weak for a detailed examination. The status of the upper and lower limbs may be determined at this time without fatiguing the patient too much. In this stage the limbs feel heavy when moved passively, and little or no muscular resistance to movement can be detected. One of the limbs—usually the upper—may be more severely affected than the other. In this case, the recovery stage of each limb is indicated on the evaluation form.

Recovery Stage 2

The basic limb synergies or some of their components now make their appearance either as weak associated reactions or on voluntary attempt to move by the patient. Components of the flexor synergy of the upper limb usually appear before components of the extensor synergy. The extent of the response, which does not necessarily result in joint movement, and the date of appearance of each response is noted in the appropriate space. Spasticity is developing but may not be very marked.

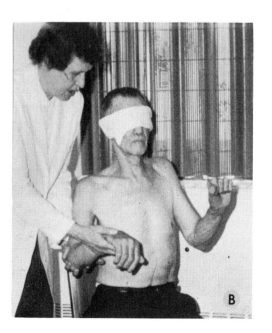

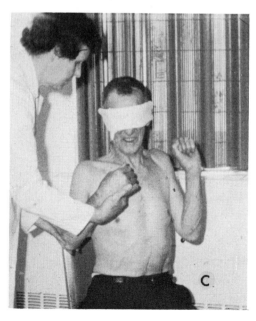

Recovery Stage 3

The basic limb synergies or some of their components are performed voluntarily and are sufficiently developed to show definite joint movements. Spasticity has increased, and during this stage it may become marked. Patients frequently remain at this stage for long periods of time and those who are severely involved may never progress beyond it.

Certain muscles, such as the pectoralis major, the pronators of the forearm, and the flexors of wrist and digits are likely to exhibit more spasticity than their antagonists; consequently, contractures may have a tendency to develop. The distribution of spasticity among the elbow muscles is more variable. At an early date, the elbow flexors may be the only ones showing spasticity. The elbow extensors usually develop spasticity later, which may or may not become as marked as that of the elbow flexors. In unusual cases, however, the spasticity of the extensor muscles may surpass that of the flexor muscles.

The status of the synergies is recorded on the evaluation form in terms of active joint range; no facilitatory measures are used. Because objective measurements of joint range would be difficult to obtain and would be disturbing to the patient, the author has settled for a subjective method, that is, an estimation of the joint range. Although such a subjective method is not ideal, it is sufficiently informative to be used clinically. Because a hemiplegia patient's ability to perform varies a great deal, not only from day to day but also from one attempt to the other, even with objective measurements the figures obtained would not be altogether reliable.

When practical, the active joint ranges may be recorded as 0, 1/4, 1/2, 3/4, or full range. At joints where such estimates are difficult, the ranges may be recorded as zero, incomplete, or complete. For elbow flexion it is convenient to record the joint angle as obtuse, 90 degrees, or acute. The date of testing is recorded at the extreme left on the evaluation form. If the test is repeated at a later date, the second column, reserved for "Active Joint Range," may be used.

The *flexor synergy* is first investigated. Figure 1-1B shows a patient performing the flexor synergy with full-range abduction and external rotation at the shoulder and with full-range elbow flexion and supination. Shoulder girdle elevation and retraction do not always appear automatically, and in such cases these movements are tested separately. The patient in Figure 1-1B uses a facilitatory head position, which is not intended to be used in testing, but if such head position is assumed spontaneously this is noted under "Remarks." Frequently, the shoulder components of abduction and external rotation are weak and replaced by hyperextension, as in Figures 1-5 and 1-6. The record of the patient in Figure 1-6 would read as follows: shoulder abduction, 0; hyperextension, $\sqrt{}$ (checked); elbow flexion, 90 degrees; supination, 1/2 range. The patient's shoulder girdle retraction appears to be complete; shoulder girdle elevation would have to be tested separately.

By demonstrating the complete flexor synergy to the patient and by having him perform first on the normal side, the examiner may ascertain whether or not the patient understands what is expected of him. A suggestion such as, "Reach up as if you were to scratch behind the ear," is frequently helpful—it gives direction to the effort. If some of the components do not respond well, these may be stressed one at a time as the patient repeats his effort. This method of emphasizing one component at a time without demanding isolated joint movements allows the patient to demonstrate his maximal capability at each joint. It also give the examiner some extra time to observe and record each joint range.

The *extensor synergy* is attempted in its entirety, as the patient is asked to reach in a forward-downward direction to touch the palm of the examiner's hand, held between the patient's knees. Figure 1-2*B* illustrates the extensor synergy with full range at all joints. The patient, however, is receiving some facilitation, which may be used for training purposes, but not in testing. If the patient does not manage to initiate the extensor synergy, the pectoralis major component (shoulder adduction in front of the body, elbow flexed) may be tested separately.

In Stage 3 the limb synergies determine the motor outcome to such an extent that flexor and extensor components do not combine. One exception, however, is commonly observed, namely, a combination of the strongest component of the extensor synergy (pectoralis major muscle) with the strongest component of the flexor synergy (elbow flexor muscles). This combination enables the patient to reach across the body toward the opposite shoulder. The muscles used are the ones that are already "overloaded" with tone, as evidenced by the reflex posture of the upper limb commonly seen in patients with spastic hemiplegia (Fig. 1-10).

The pronator muscles of the forearm are frequently equally "overloaded," particularly if the hemiparesis is of long standing. If this is so, these muscles, although they belong to the extensor synergy, may fail to yield when the flexor synergy is willed. In such patients, external rotation of the shoulder is also weak or lacking (Fig. 1-8). A wrist drop resulting from spasticity of the wrist flexor muscles is likewise conducive to the pronated position because the weight of the hand tends to maintain pronation (Fig. 1-7). But when hyperextension replaces abduction, the supination component regularly appears (Figs. 1-5 and 1-6).

Recovery Stage 4

When the patient progesses beyond Stage 3, spasticity begins to decrease, and some movement combinations that deviate from the basic limb synergies become available. Three combinations that are comparatively easy to master have been selected to represent Stage 4. These three movements are further discussed in Chapter 3.

1. Placing the Hand behind the Body (Fig. 3-8A). This movement necessitates the activation of a number of posterior muscles that are not component parts of either synergy, such as the rhomboid muscles as downward rotators of the scapula, the latissimus dorsi, and the teres major muscles. Simultaneously, the pectoralis major muscle must be inhibited. The movement is not as difficult as it may appear at first, because it can utilize first a modified flexor synergy then a modified extensor synergy.

2. Elevation of the Arm to a Forward-Horizontal Position. Successful completion of this movement is a sign that the originally strong linkage between the pectoralis major and the triceps muscles is declining. For a passing grade, the elbow must be kept fully extended.

3. Pronation-supination, elbows at 90 degrees. The movement is performed bilaterally so that a comparison of the two sides can be made. Bilateral performance has several advantages and is employed for the investigation even though, possibly, the testing rule of "no facilitation" may be violated (Fig. 2-3). Range of motion, not speed, is empasized. The elbows are kept close to the sides of the body, for if shoulder abduction is allowed, particularly in the presence of a wrist drop, the forearm will fall into pronation by the action of gravity. The tendency on the affected side to move the elbow away from the body to aid in pronation is seen in Figure 2-3*B*.

Recovery Stage 5

A relative independence of the basic limb synergies characterizes this stage, and spasticity is waning. More difficult movement combinations can be performed, and

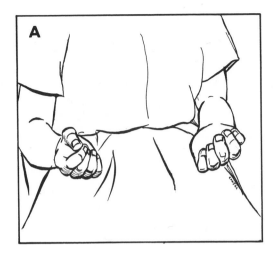

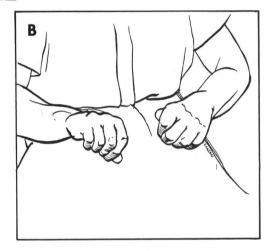

FIGURE 2-3. Pronation and supination of forearms by 58-year-old patient with left-sided hemiparesis, 10 months following a cerebral vascular accident. (Drawn from frames of a motion picture.) **A.** On the right (normal) side pronation has begun, while on the left (affected) side the forearm remains supinated. **B.** On the left side, abduction and internal rotation of the shoulder has been used to aid in pronation.

certain individual joint movements may succeed, but the patient may have to concentrate intensely on some of the tasks. Easier movement combinations, e.g., those representative of Stage 4, are performed in a more effortless manner. The borderline between Stages 4 and 5 is difficult to draw because the gaining of control of the var-

ious movement combinations is a gradual process. Three movements have been chosen to represent Stage 5.

1. Arm-Raising to a Side-Horizontal Position. The movement starts with the arm hanging relaxed at the side of the body. The arm is raised laterally with the elbow extended and the forearm pronated as in Figure 2-4B. To correctly execute this movement, two components of the flexor synergy (retraction of the shoulder girdle and abduction of the shoulder) must combine with two components of the extensor synergy (extension of the elbow and pronation of the forearm), and the pectoralis major muscle must become disassociated from the triceps muscle. This movement can only be performed properly when the basic limb synergies have lost their influence to the extent that voluntary impulses prevail.

The patient in Figure 2-4A (shown 4 weeks following a cerebral vascular accident) had gained control of the basic limb synergies and could also perform the three movements listed for Stage 4. When requested to raise the arm laterally to a horizontal position, she could not do so in the prescribed manner. She attempted to solve the problem by first performing a typical flexor synergy with complete range of abduction and external rotation of the shoulder, flexion of the elbow and supination of the forearm. From this position she endeavored to extend the elbow but was unsuccessful because the synergy influence could not be overcome—the elbow flexor muscles would not release their contraction, and the forearm remained supinated. In Figure 2-4B (6 months following the acute episode) the synergy influence had disappeared, and arm-raising laterally to the horizontal position was performed in a normal manner. The exact time that this ability was acquired was not documented by motion pictures. It occurred during the period that the patient was treated in an out-patient clinic.

46

2. Arm-Raising Forward and Overhead.

The first portion of this movement (elevation of the arm forward to the horizontal) was tested in Stage 4, so that if the patient is going to score at all in Stage 5 the arm must be raised above the horizontal. For full credit, the movement must be performed with the elbow extended and must closely resemble the corrresponding movement on the uninvolved side, as in Figure 2-5*B* and *C*.

The patient in Figure 2-5*A* makes an effort to raise the arm overhead, but the movement is arrested half way up. She is again using the flexor synergy that she attempts to adapt to the task before her. Five months later, the synergy influence has been overcome and the movement is well under control.

3. Pronation-Supination, Elbow Extended.

The movement may be performed bilaterally or unilaterally. No attempt is made to isolate pronation-supination of the forearm from internal-external rotation of the shoulder. The patient is asked to turn the palms up and down alternately, and if this is done satisfactorily increase in speed may be attempted. The test may be given with the arms in the forward-horizontal or side-horizontal position. The latter position is likely to be more difficult as long as some influence of the synergies remains. Such influence was no longer present in the case of the patient seen in Figure 2-6, 6 months following a cerebral vascular accident.

Recovery Stage 6.

Isolated joint movements are now freely performed, that is, as well on the affected as on the unaffected side. In general, movements are well coordinated and appear normal or near normal. The basic movement synergies no longer interfere with the performance of a variety of move-

FIGURE 2-4. This patient, age 52, has a right-sided hemiparesis resulting from a thrombosis of the left middle cerebral artery. (Frames of a motion picture.) *A*. Four weeks after the acute episode, because of synergy influence, the patient was unable to abduct the affected arm laterally to a horizontal position (see text). *B*. Six months after the acute episode, arm-raising laterally was performed in the prescribed manner.

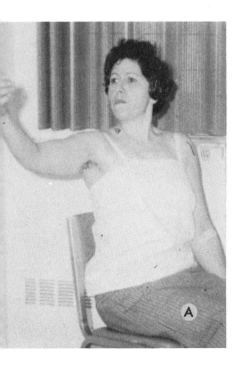

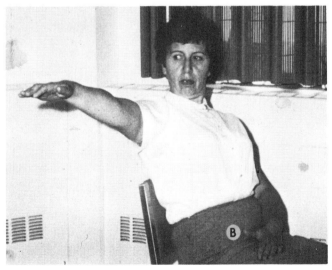

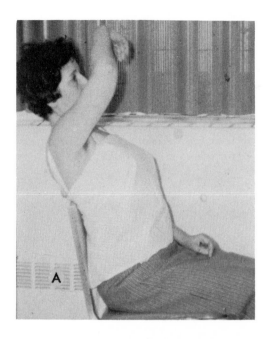

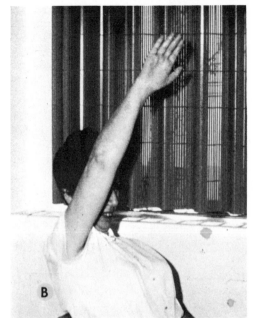

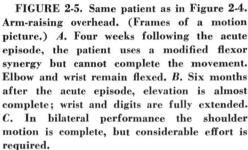

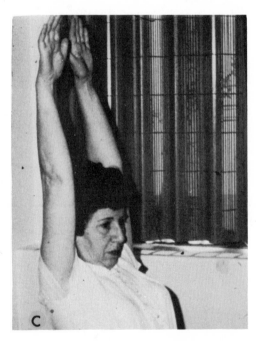

FIGURE 2-5. Same patient as in Figure 2-4. Arm-raising overhead. (Frames of a motion picture.) *A.* Four weeks following the acute episode, the patient uses a modified flexor synergy but cannot complete the movement. Elbow and wrist remain flexed. *B.* Six months after the acute episode, elevation is almost complete; wrist and digits are fully extended. *C.* In bilateral performance the shoulder motion is complete, but considerable effort is required.

ment combinations, but under close examination some awkwardness may be observed. Spasticity cannot be demonstrated by passive movements of the limbs, but active movements with increasing speed may reveal an interference on the affected side, which may or may not be called spasticity.

Speed Tests

The speed tests found on page 2 of the evaluation form may be given to assess spasticity during any one of the recovery stages, provided the patient possesses sufficient range of active motion to carry out the movements as prescribed. These tests are particularly applicable to Stages 4

to 6. For purpose of comparison, both the unaffected and the affected sides are tested. Because the movements chosen closely resemble the flexor and the extensor synergies, a patient need not be independent of the synergies to participate. The two movements studied are:

1. Hand from lap to chin, requiring complete range of flexion of the elbow (Fig. 2-7)

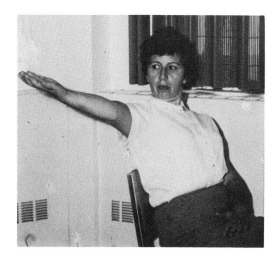

FIGURE 2-6. Same patient as in Figures 2-4 and 2-5. With the arm on the affected side raised laterally, 6 months after a cerebral vascular accident the patient experiences no difficulty in turning the palm up and down while keeping elbow, wrist, and fingers extended. The palm-down position is seen in Figure 2-4B. (Frame of a motion picture.)

2. Hand from lap to opposite knee, requiring full range of extension of the elbow (Fig. 2-8)

The patient is seated on a sturdy chair without arm rests. He leans against the back of the chair, keeping the head erect. The hand of the limb to be tested rests in the lap, fist lightly closed. For the first test, the forearm is half way between pronation and supination so that when the hand touches the chin, the chin fits into the open space between the thumb and the index finger. In the second test, the forearm is pronated. The movements are well defined because the fist must touch a definite mark at the end of each movement path. A stop watch is used and the number of full strokes (back and forth movements) completed in five seconds is recorded, first on the normal, then on the affected side. If the speed is slow, as would be the case when spasticity is marked, "half-strokes" are counted as well.

These two speed tests give information concerning spasticity of the flexor and extensor muscles of the elbow. If more

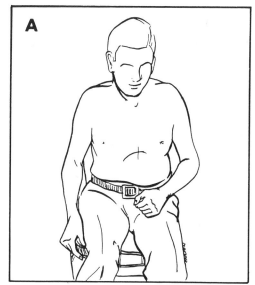

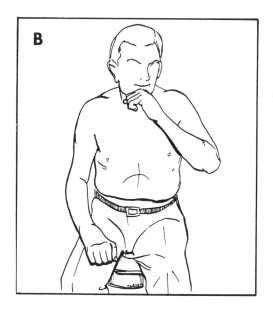

FIGURE 2-7. Speed test, hand from lap to chin. A. Starting position. The ulnar side of the hand is held in the lap, close to the groin. B. The hand is brought up to the chin and returned to the starting position with as much speed as possible (see text).

complete assessment of spasticity is desired, other muscle groups would have to be tested also.

MOTOR TESTS: HAND

A different approach to the evaluation of hand function from that employed for the

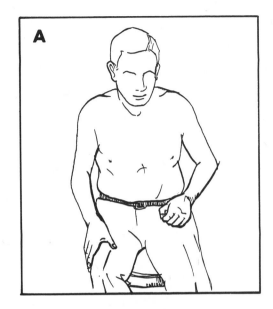

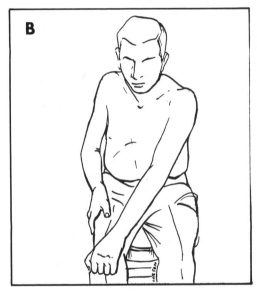

FIGURE 2-8. Speed test, hand from lap to opposite knee. *A.* Starting position. The fist, palmar side down, is held in the lap near the groin. The patient leans against the back of the chair. *B.* The fist reaches out to touch the knee on the opposite side and returns to the starting position with as much speed as possible (see text).

limb as a whole has been found desirable because the return of hand function may not in every respect parallel the six recovery stages outlined above. As an example, patients have been seen who show com-

paratively speedy return of hand function although more proximal joints are poorly controlled. However, in general the return of hand function, like that of the rest of the limb, proceeds from flaccidity to spasticity, then decrease of, and eventually cessation of, spasticity—provided that progress continues. This is in accordance with the findings by Twitchell (1951).

Wrist Stabilization for Grasp

The ability to stabilize the wrist in extension during voluntary fist closure is examined in two positions: with the elbow extended and with the elbow flexed. Under normal circumstances, wrist stabilization is automatic, but after a stroke it is often lacking.

As long as the synergies are dominant, the wrist has a tendency to flex when the elbow flexes. A strong association between elbow flexion and wrist flexion is illustrated in Figure 2-9. With the elbow extended, satisfactory wrist fixation appears automatically on fist closure. But when the elbow is flexed and the patient attempts to close the fist, the wrist remains flexed. The fist closure seen on the *normal* side in Figure 2-9*B* and *C* ("imitation synkinesis") indicates that the patient makes a strong effort to close the fist on the affected side. Note that in Figure 2-9*A* the normal hand does not close; apparently strong effort was not required when the elbow was extended.

In Figure 2-9*D*, the same patient, 6 months following the cerebral vascular accident, demonstrates wrist fixation for grasp with elbow flexed; synergy influence was no longer present at that time. No imitation synkinesis appears on the normal side.

Wrist Flexion and Extension, Fist Closed

This movement tests a patient's control of wrist flexion and extension with an

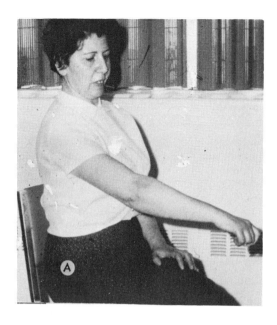

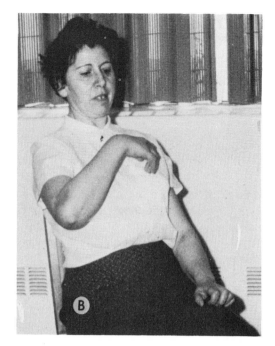

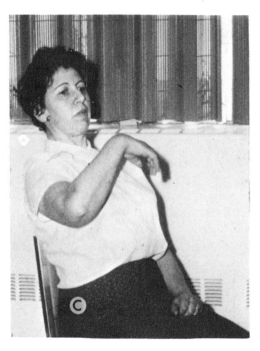

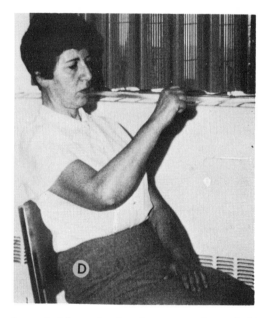

FIGURE 2-9. Patient with right-sided hemiparesis (As shown in Figures 2-4, 2-5, and 2-6), 7 weeks after a cerebral vascular accident (*A, B, C*) and 6 months after-stroke (*D*). (Frames from a motion picture.) *A.* Fist closure with the elbow extended is accompanied by wrist extension. *B.* When the elbow flexes, the wrist also flexes; fist closure cannot be accomplished. *C.* The patient makes an unsuccessful effort to extend the wrist; the effort is reflected in the extended position of head, neck, and trunk. *D.* Elbow flexion no longer interferes with wrist fixation for grasp.

object held in the hand, a control needed for many skilled activities. Only a moderate range of wrist flexion is required because full range of flexion is seldom utilized in functional activities.

Wrist Circumduction

If the hand can be moved smoothly in a circling fashion, recovery is well advanced. When examining this movement, the patient's forearm is stabilized in pronation to prevent a combination of pronation-supination movements and wrist movements, a combination which many normal individuals tend to utilize when requested to perform circumduction.

Wrist circumduction requires a high degree of coordination and is much more difficult than wrist stabilization for grasp. For testing intermediate stages, isolated wrist movements of radial and ulnar flexion may be recorded, but these are not included on the evaluation form.

Prehension

On the remainder of page 2 of the evaluation form, the patient's ability to open and close the hand (mass grasp and mass extension) and to utilize various types of prehensions in handling objects is recorded.

Prehension types are listed in order of their difficulty, beginning with *hook grasp*, for holding on to the handles of a handbag placed in the hand, and ending with *spherical grasp*, used in grasping a ball or an apple. Release of grasp is not required for the hook grasp test, but for the other types of prehension the object must not only be grasped but also released.

Lateral prehension is used to grasp a small object, such as a card, between the radial side of the index and the thumb. *Palmar prehension* necessitates opposition of the thumb to one or more fingers, a type of prehension commonly used to grasp small objects and for many skilled hand activities (Fig. 2-10). *Cylindrical grasp* is used to pick up and hold larger objects, such as a jar or a mug (Fig. 2-11). *Spherical grasp* is listed last because in addition to grasp and release of a ball (Fig. 2-12), the patient's ability to catch and throw a ball may be investigated. These latter activities are indeed difficult for patients with hemiplegia because they require a rapid fist closure and rapid release and coordinated control of the entire limb. In all prehension types the performances on the two sides are compared and the patient's handedness—right or left—is taken into consideration.

Individual Thumb Movements

For the sake of standardization, the patient's hands rest in the lap, ulnar side down. The two thumb movements to be investigated may then be explained to the patient as "up and down" and "side-to-side" movements. The normal side always performs first, then the affected side.

Individual Finger Movements

These are briefly described in the appropriate space. Isolated control of flexion and extension at the metacarpophalangeal joints of the index and the middle finger may be expected before radial and ulnar abduction can be performed. It is particularly important to pay attention to radial abduction of the index finger to counteract the tendency to ulnar abduction commonly observed during finger extension, and to prevent atrophy of the muscles in the interosseous space between the thumb and the index finger.

If an attempt is made to correlate restoration of hand function with the sequential recovery stages outlined for the limb as a whole, the classification, approximately, would be as follows:

Stage 1. Flaccidity
Stage 2. Little or no active finger flexion
Stage 3. Mass grasp; use of hook grasp but no release; no voluntary finger extension; possibly, reflex extension of digits
Stage 4. Lateral prehension, release by thumb movement; semivoluntary finger extension, small range
Stage 5. Palmar prehension, possibly cylindrical and spherical grasp, awkwardly performed and with limited functional use; voluntary

mass extension of digits, variable range

Stage 6. All prehensile types under control; skills improving; full-range voluntary extension of digits; individual finger movements present, less accurate than on opposite side

MOTOR TESTS:
TRUNK AND LOWER LIMB

For practical reasons, the patient is tested first in the supine position, then sitting, then standing; finally, if the patient is ambulatory, his gait is analyzed. These tests, as outlined on page 3 of the evaluation form, are largely self-explanatory, hence every item need not be discussed here.

Because it is important to assess the behavior of the lower limb in different body postures, the space allotted to the supine position on the evaluation form is rather limited. The status of the flexor and extensor synergies and of hip abduction and adduction must be very briefly noted. As an aid to the examiner, a standardized procedure for testing may be outlined on a separate sheet. The sitting and standing tests give additional information concerning the status of the limb synergies.

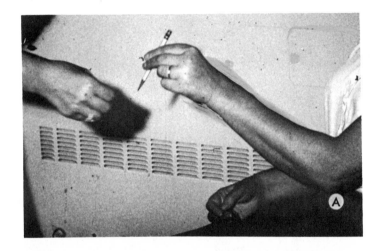

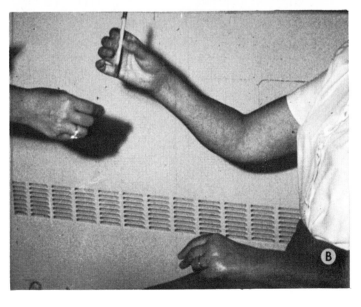

FIGURE 2-10. Palmar prehension by same patient with right-sided hemiparesis, 6 months following a stroke. A pencil is handed to the patient without instructions how to grasp it. *A.* Normal hand. *B.* Affected hand. Palmar prehension appears to be accomplished by mass flexion of fingers and opposition of the thumb. Note its resemblance to tip prehension.

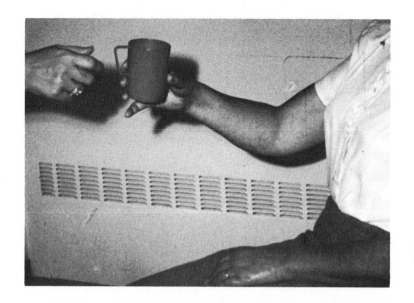

FIGURE 2-11. Cylindrical grasp, same patient. Grasp is functionally satisfactory, but imperfect.

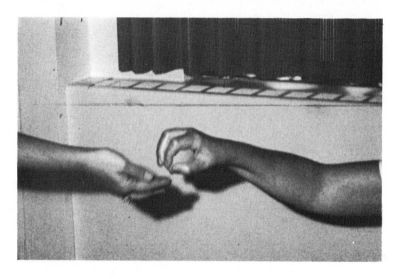

FIGURE 2-12. Spherical grasp, same patient. With the hand stationary, the ball was released with ease. Throwing and catching were awkward.

The return of function of the lower limb in terms of recovery stages may be expressed as follows:

Stage 1. Flaccidity

Stage 2. Minimal voluntary movements of the lower limb

Stage 3. Hip-knee-ankle flexion in sitting and standing

Stage 4. Sitting, knee flexion beyond 90 degrees with the foot sliding backward on the floor; voluntary dorsiflexion of the ankle without lifting the foot off the floor

Stage 5. Standing, isolated nonweight-bearing knee flexion, hip extended or nearly extended; standing, isolated dorsiflexion of the ankle, knee extended, heel forward in a position of a short step

Stage 6. Standing, hip abduction beyond range obtained from elevation of the pelvis; sitting, reciprocal action of the inner and outer hamstring muscles, resulting in inward and outward rotation of the leg at the knee, combined with inversion and eversion of the ankle

The reciprocal contraction of the semitendinosus and the biceps femoris muscles may be verified by palpation of their tendons at the knee. Such *reciprocal* action, as distinguished from their *synergistic* action during knee flexion, indicates a high degree of restoration of function of the neuromuscular system; their reciprocal action has therefore been chosen to represent Stage 6.

When examining a patient it is not unusual to find that the upper and the lower limbs belong to different recovery stages. The lower limb is frequently less affected than the upper, but the reverse also occurs.

The patient's ambulatory status is then recorded, and if the patient is sufficiently advanced, the examiner proceeds with a gait analysis, noting the deviations observed at ankle, knee, and hip in the stance phase and the swing phase. Familiarity with the material contained in Chapter 4 and with the detailed gait analysis form (Chart 2) is essential for this portion of the examination.

ABBREVIATED EVALUATION FORMS

There has been frequent need for a short form to be used when a less detailed sensory and motor appraisal is required.

With the long form as a model, several short ones have been prepared, but these are not included here. The author believes that the short forms so far prepared are not altogether satisfactory. They are less informative with respect to the recovery status of a patient and his progress. Furthermore, they do not clearly reveal the rationale for patient evaluation and therapeutic procedures, hence are less suitable for teaching purposes.

These statements are not made to discourage experimentation with shorter forms. Such experimentation is desirable, even if a form thus produced may not prove universally acceptable because, at the present time, requirements vary greatly at different institutions.

REFERENCES

Lovett, R. W. *The Treatment of Infantile Paralysis.* 2nd ed. Philadelphia, Blakiston, 1917, p. 136.

Reynolds, G., Archibald, K. C., Brunnstrom, S., and Thompson, N. Preliminary report on neuromuscular function testing of the upper extremity in adult hemiplegic patients. *Arch. Phys. Med.* 39:303, 1958.

Twitchell, T. E. The restoration of motor function following hemiplegia in man. *Brain* 47:443, 1951.

3

Training Procedures

The information contained in Chapters 1 and 2 has been supplied to acquaint the student with the motor behavior and the sequential recovery stages of patients with hemiplegia. This information, together with the student's background knowledge in neurophysiology and neuropathology and his familiarity with the abstracts in the Appendix, should materially contribute to his understanding of the rationale for the training procedures to be outlined.

PSYCHOLOGICAL ASPECTS

A constructive patient-therapist relationship requires that the patient gain confidence in the physical therapist's ability to deal with the problems at hand. The physical therapist, too, must have confidence—in his own knowledge, skills, and judgment. The more the physical therapist understands the patient's sensorimotor difficulties, the better is he equipped to direct the training procedures. Such understanding is almost immediately sensed by the patient. A tacit partnership between instructor and patient develops, and the stage is set for a cooperative adventure. Conversely, if such understanding is lacking, the patient feels ill at ease and is reluctant to make the effort required of him.

It would be most inappropriate to expect the patient to learn control of isolated joint movements at a time when the synergy influence is strong. Not only would such a demand be without success, but fundamental learning principles would be violated. Repeated failures by the patient to carry out the tasks demanded of him would lead to frustration and disappointment, and sooner or later motivation would suffer. The patient's confidence in the physical therapist would become undermined, for the patient intuitively would feel that the therapist should know better than to demand the impossible.

The training sessions must be planned in such a manner that *only those tasks which the patient can master, or almost master,* will be demanded of him. Success, no matter how small, is an important reward —it maintains interest and boosts motivation.

At the first meeting with the patient, the physical therapist must show a genuine and unhurried interest in the patient's welfare, but he must refrain from asking too many questions about the onset and course of the illness. If he has read the patient's history in advance he is already oriented in that respect, and most questions are unnecessary. For the purpose of getting acquainted, he chats for a short while with the patient, then introduces the therapeutic procedures, but only gradually. It is better to do too little than too much during the first session. The physical therapist must carefully observe the patient's reactions and attitudes because his observations will serve as a guide for the next session. An optimistic and matter-of-fact attitude is usually appreciated by the patient, but no promises and predictions in regard to his recovery should be made.

The technical skills that the physical therapists needs and the judgment that he must possess in dealing with patients with hemiplegia can only be gained by clinical experience. However, it is hoped that the procedures offered in the training chapters will serve their purpose, namely, to introduce the student to a neurophysiological approach to movement therapy, an approach that has many psychological implications as well as technical aspects.

BED POSTURE AND BED EXERCISES

BED POSTURE

Attention is given to the patient's bed posture while the flaccid condition prevails and the limbs may be placed in the most favorable positions without interference by spastic muscles. This is often the responsibility of the nurse since the physical therapist may not be called in to see the patient at such early date. It is therefore essential that nurses be informed about the influence of the basic limb synergies on the bed posture of patients with hemiplegia.

Flexor Posture, Lower Limb. Bed patients who have been unsupervised for some time tend to assume a lower limb posture consisting of external rotation and abduction of the hip and flexion of the knee on the affected side. Such posture appears to be caused in part by mechanical and in part by neurological factors: mechanical, because the weight distribution in a flaccid lower limb causes external rotation of the hip, and because the weight of the bed clothes on the limb tends to maintain the described position; neurological, because the joint positions at hip and knee correspond to those of the flexor synergy. When this synergy makes its appearance, muscular tension in the flexor and abductor muscles of the hip contributes to the hip posture mentioned; knee flexion appears simultaneously.

Extensor Posture, Lower Limb. At a date when the extensor synergy of the lower limb is fully developed, a different limb posture may appear. At that time, spasticity in the extensor muscles often exceeds that of the flexor muscles. The ensuing posture becomes characterized by extension and adduction of the hip, extension of the knee, and plantar flexion of the ankle. When severe spasticity in the adductor muscles is present, the patient may get into a habit of placing the normal foot under the affected leg; this allows the affected limb to adduct further so that a crossed-limb posture results.

Recommended Bed Posture, Lower Limb. When the patient lies on his back, the following bed posture—to alternate with a lateral position—is recommended: slight hip and knee flexion, maintained by a small pillow under the knee; lateral support of the knee to prevent abduction and external rotation of the hip; and proper support of the bed clothes to prevent them from pressing on the foot.

The flexed hip-knee position is recommended because knee flexion, even in a small range, has an inhibitory effect on the extensor muscles of knee and ankle, thus counteracting the development of excessive uncontrolled tension in these muscles, a tension that would prove to hinder ambulation.

However, if the flexion synergy predominates over the extensor synergy in the lower limb, the flexed hip-knee position in bed is unsuitable and the knee must be kept extended. Obviously, the choice of bed posture must be determined on an individual basis. (A patient exhibiting marked predominance of flexion in the lower limb is discussed in Chapter 5 and illustrated in Figs. 5-5 and 5-6.)

Recommended Bed Posture, Upper Limb. The upper limb is supported on a pillow in a position that is comfortable for the patient. Abduction of the humerus with respect to the scapula must be avoided as it deprives the shoulder joint of the stabilizing action of the lower portion of the glenoid fossa on the humeral head and slackens the superior portion of the capsule, thus predisposing to a downward subluxation of the humeral head (Basmajian, 1966). In handling the patient, traction on the affected arm is avoided and the patient is instructed to use his normal hand to support the affected arm when moving around in bed. (The role of muscles in preventing subluxation of the shoulder joint is discussed later in this chapter.)

BED EXERCISES

Passive and Active Assisted Movements. For the choice of bed exercises, the physical therapist must be guided by instructions received from the physician in charge, by information found in the patient's record and by his own good judgment. Passive motions of the limbs are first carried out, and then developed into active assisted motions. The program is expanded to include head, neck, and trunk movements. The patient is also shown how to move around in bed while protecting the affected arm; he learns to sit up and to turn to the side-lying position.

Turning from Supine to Side-Lying Position. Most patients find it easier to turn toward the affected side because this requires little or no activity of the paretic limbs. The affected arm is placed close to the body, and in turning the patient rolls over the affected arm, to which he seldom objects unless it causes pain. Turning toward the unaffected side is illustrated in Figure 3-1. This turn is more difficult because it requires active participation by the affected limbs. The patient in the illustration is unable to control her left arm, hence uses the normal hand to elevate it. The affected lower limb is brought up into partial flexion and, if necessary, is momentarily stabilized in this position by the therapist. Figure 3-1A shows the starting position from which the patient attempts to turn over by swinging the arms and the left knee across the body. The limb movements substantially aid in turning the upper body and the pelvis, respectively. In Figure 3-1B the turn has been completed, guided by the therapist. When control improves, the turn is carried out as one continuous movement from the supine to the side-lying position.

Prone position for "unlocking" flexed joints. The face-down position is unsuitable for many elderly stroke patients who find that the position is uncomfortable and restricts their breathing. Other stroke patients, however, and children with cerebral palsy do not object to turning face down, and manipulations recommended by Fay (1954) may then be utilized to

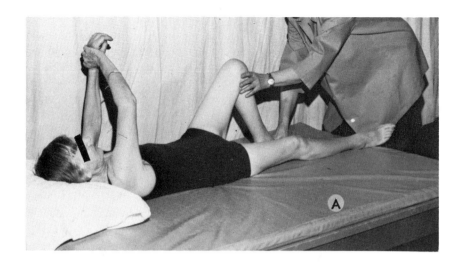

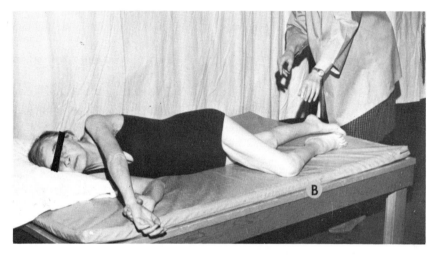

FIGURE 3-1. Turning from supine to side-lying position (see text). The patient, age 71, has a left-sided hemiparesis of 3 months' duration, resulting from a thrombosis of the right middle cerebral artery. *A.* Starting position. *B.* Movement has been completed.

"unlock" joints kept in flexion as a result of spasticity.

For manipulations of the upper limb, an adult patient lies close to the edge of the treatment table, his head rotated toward the affected side. The flexed elbow is elevated until the upper arm is horizontal, then the shoulder is inward rotated and by means of a sweeping movement the dorsum of the hand is brought to a position over the buttocks. In primitive animal locomotion, Fay (1954) states, the latter limb position constitutes the end of the flexion stroke, hence flexion tension diminishes and disappears in preparation for the extension stroke. The manipulation then continues and the arm is brought in an outward and forward direction, which rep-resents the extension stroke. The entire movement follows a roundabout path that resembles a swimmer's crawl stroke.

TRUNK, NECK, AND LIMB TRAINING IN SITTING POSITION

As soon as feasible, the sitting rather than the supine position is used for training. First, in the sitting position the patient has an opportunity to improve his trunk balance and to gain control of simple trunk movements. Second, if the therapist sits facing the patient, communication between the two is made easy. A face-to-face encounter is valuable in dealing with all types of patients, and it is indispensable if the patient is aphasic. Third, trunk movements guided by the therapist may be employed to evoke or facilitate certain arm movements over which the patient may have no voluntary control. Fourth, orientation of the upper limb to the erect position at an early date is essential because so many important functional activities are performed in sitting; a direct carry-over of arm control from the supine to the sitting position does not necessarily take place.

SITTING TRUNK BALANCE
(see also Chapter 5)

Many patients with hemiplegia have good trunk balance soon after a stroke, but others have a tendency to deviate from the normal symmetrical trunk posture in sitting. This tendency may be evident when the patient sits in a wheelchair, but for a closer examination and for training in trunk balance, the patient is transferred to a sturdy chair without arm rests.

The Listing Phenomenon. To observe the listing phenomenon, the patient is first assisted into a symmetrical sitting posture away from the back of the chair. When the assistance is withdrawn, the patient's trunk begins to list toward the affected side, as if drawn by a magnet, and if the listing is not checked, a fall may result.

The patient in Figure 3-2 regularly listed toward the affected side when not observed. At the time the photograph was taken, she was apparently aware of the tendency and braced herself by grasping the side of the chair with her right hand.

It is rather peculiar that the listing should occur toward the *affected* side because once the center of gravity of the upper portion of the body has been shifted slightly toward that side, the trunk muscles on the *unaffected* side would be the ones required to check the movement, yet these muscles fail to bring the trunk back to the midline. A further discussion of this phenomenon is found in Chapter 5.

The statement that trunk listing occurs toward the affected side is not intended to imply that this is universally so. Occasionally, a slight trunk deviation toward the unaffected side may be observed. This deviation, however, appears as a rather stationary posture, not as a gradually increasing trunk listing. Possibly, trunk deviation toward the unaffected side may be explained as a compensatory habit which the patient has acquired to avoid listing in the opposite direction.

Evoking Balancing Responses. For the purpose of eliciting balancing responses, the sitting trunk posture is deliberately disturbed in forward-backward and side-to-side directions. To avoid frightening the patient, the procedure is first explained to her. She is pushed out of balance, first gently, then more vigorously. In Figure 3-2B and C, the "push" was exaggerated. Note how the patient supports the affected arm to protect the shoulder joint. This arm posture also prevents the patient from grasping the side of the chair with the normal hand. The balancing responses at this time are not automatic, but eventually the patient may be given a light push without warning. Disturbing the balance in the direction toward which the patient tends to list is considered particularly important. In the illustration two physical therapists are engaged in the game, but one person standing behind the patient can also safely handle the situation.

TRUNK BENDING FORWARD
AND OBLIQUELY FORWARD

These movements are here called "trunk bending" because the patient is told to bend forward, but they would perhaps better be referred to as "trunk inclination," as they take place mainly at the hips and consist of a movement of the trunk with respect to the thighs, with little or no ventroflexion of the vertebral column.

The patient sits in a straight-back chair and supports the affected arm as before. For the first trials, and as long as needed, the therapist guides the trunk and arm movements by holding his hands under the patient's elbows (Fig. 3-3). If the patient's trunk balance is poor the therapist may use his own knees to stabilize the patient's knees, because the knee on the affected side has a tendency to fall out into abduction. In the case of the patient illustrated, such stabilization was not required.

As the trunk inclines forward, the therapist guides the patient's arms in order to attain glenohumeral and scapular motions. Because the serratus anterior muscle may not be functioning on the affected side and the antagonistic muscles may be tight, the instructor gently assists the forward movement of the scapula if he manages to reach the medial border of the scapula; traction on the arm should be avoided.

The movement is more demanding in terms of trunk control if it is performed in oblique directions, forward to the left and forward to the right. When the therapist guides these movements it is suggested that he assume the standing position, because he can then follow through more thoroughly and he has the patient's balance better under control.

The forward inclination of the trunk, whether straight or oblique, calls upon the two-joint hamstring muscles to act as hip extensors and is employed as a preliminary step for evoking responses of these muscle.

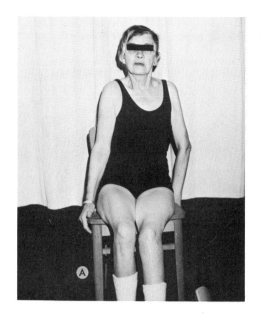

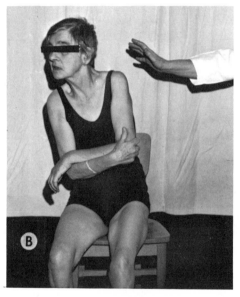

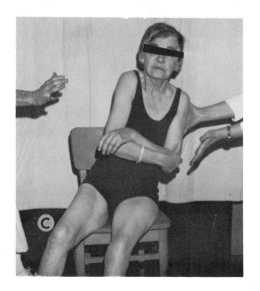

FIGURE 3-2. Sitting trunk balance, same patient. *A.* The listing phenomenon. Patient is aware of a listing tendency and grasps the side of the chair with her right hand. When unobserved, listing became marked. *B* and *C.* Balancing responses are evoked (see text).

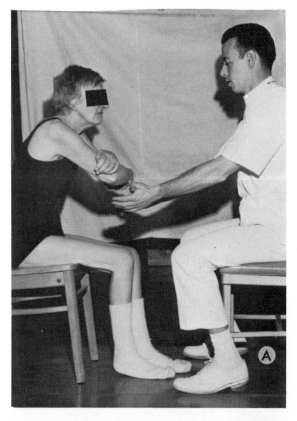

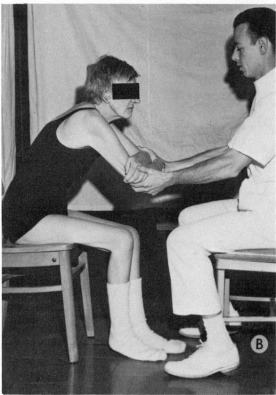

as knee flexors. This procedure is further discussed in Chapter 5.

TRUNK ROTATION

The patient supports his affected arm as before and the therapist sits facing the patient and guides the movement. In some cases the therapist may stand behind the patient to emphasize rotation (Fig. 3-4). Trunk rotation is first performed gently and within small range, then the range is gradually increased. Throughout the movement the patient looks straight ahead, which results not only in movement of the upper body with respect to the pelvis, but also in rotation of the trunk with respect to the head and neck. A certain amount of neck mobilization is thus obtained without the patient noticing it. Additional head rotation takes place if the head rotates maximally to the right while the trunk rotates toward the left, and vice versa.

It might be confusing to the patient to be told to rotate the trunk to one side and the head to the other side, and therefore such instructions are avoided. Head movements in the desired directions may evolve almost automatically if the therapist demonstrates the movements and encourages the patient to "look over the shoulder." If trunk rotation is guided slowly and rhythmically, the patient need not pay any attention to the direction of this movement, and then the instructions, "Look right, look left," may be given in a rhythm corresponding to the trunk movement. Should confusion arise, the patient is told to forget about the head movement and look straight ahead.

In the neutral position, before trunk rotation begins, the patient's arms are close to the body and relatively relaxed, except

FIGURE 3-3. Trunk inclination forward, same patient with left-sided hemiparesis. *A.* The forward movement is guided by the physical therapist who supports the patient's two elbows. *B.* The return movement is performed without support.

for the upward pressure on the elbow on the affected side. As the trunk rotates, the patient maintains a firm grip around the affected elbow, and the arms swing rhythmically from side to side; the principal movements are shoulder abduction on one side and shoulder adduction on the other side. Each time the movement is reversed the arms are lowered to the starting position before the trunk rotates toward the other side. The affected arm may have to be carried along passively for a number of days, but some active participation by its muscles may be expected before long. A total trunk-neck-arm pattern evolves. The shoulder components of the flexor and extensor synergies are evoked alternately and are initiated, or reinforced, by the tonic lumbar and tonic neck reflexes. If the linkage between synergy components is strong, trunk rotation may evoke a complete extensor synergy (including full-range elbow extension) in patients who cannot voluntarily perform any part of the extensor synergy. Such extension occurs when the trunk rotates toward the normal side and the head rotates toward the affected side.

HEAD AND NECK MOVEMENTS

Restrictions in the range of head and neck movements are common among elderly individuals, and stroke patients are no exceptions. Some increased flexibility of the cervical spine may be obtained from flexion and extension movements, from side bending and rotation movements. Manual "spine lengthening" by traction on the head may be included.

Neuromuscular control of head and neck movements within the available range is usually present following a stroke, and this

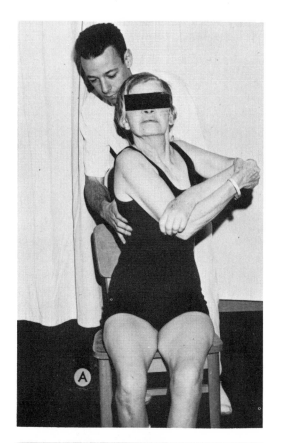

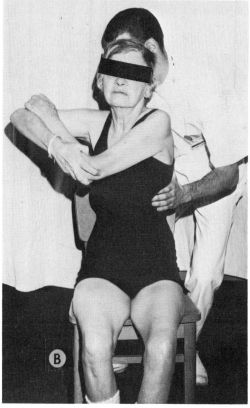

FIGURE 3-4. Trunk rotation, same patient. Note the manner in which the patient supports the affected arm. To obtain increased range of rotation, the physical therapist guides the movement. *A.* Rotation toward affected side. *B.* Rotation toward normal side.

control may be utilized to facilitate shoulder girdle movements over which the patient may have little or no control. As an example, the upper trapezius muscle may be observed to contract when resistance is given to head side-bending, yet the patient may be unable to use the same muscle if he attempts to elevate the shoulder girdle.

Because in the following method the physical therapist's hands will be occupied in providing resistance, the patient's affected arm is placed on a nearby table or treatment plinth in an abducted position with the elbow flexed and the forearm and hand supported. The physical therapist holds one hand over the acromioclavicular region, the other hand on the side of the patient's head, which is inclined toward the shoulder, and gives the commands "Hold," or "Don't let me pull your head away from your shoulder." If an isometric or lengthening contraction is successful, it is followed by a shortening contraction. During this procedure resistance is given on the shoulder as well as on the head; the patient's attention is focused on the head movement and he experiences the sensation of "holding." Thereafter, the patient concentrates his effort on holding the shoulder "close to the ear," and pressure on the shoulder is emphasized. The tension in the shoulder elevator muscles, which has been built up during resisted head side-bending, may thus make voluntary shoulder elevation materialize.

RANGE OF MOTION AT SHOULDER
(Preliminary Approach)

A definite relationship appears to exist between shoulder pain and the stretching of spastic muscles about the shoulder joint. If the patient anticipates pain, muscular tension increases, and pain on passive movement is aggravated. Mobilization of the shoulder joint without forceful stretching of tense muscles is therefore desirable.

Patients who experience pain if the physical therapist attempts to move the arm with respect to the trunk may have no complaints during trunk movements which, if properly guided, result in a considerable amount of shoulder mobilization. For example, when the trunk inclines forward, the elbows supported by the therapist move in a forward direction, and the greater the trunk inclination, the more shoulder range is obtained (Fig. 3-3). Similarly, trunk rotation is accompanied by alternate abduction and adduction movements (Fig. 3-4). In this indirect way, painless shoulder movements are obtained. The absence of pain may be explained as follows.

First, the patient feels secure because he himself supports the affected arm and is thus able to protect the shoulder. Second, his attention is focused on trunk movements, and whatever shoulder movements occur are hardly noticed by the patient. Third, during trunk rotation both neck and lumbar reflexes play a part in causing an alternate increase and decrease in the tension of the pectoralis major muscle on the affected side. When tension in this muscle is decreased, abduction can proceed in larger range without resistance by the muscle and without pain. When the shoulder abductor muscles begin to participate actively during trunk rotation, additional release of tension in the pectoralis major muscle may be expected, and painless abduction is further enhanced.

Once the patient is confident that no pain is going to be produced, active assisted movements of the arm with respect to the trunk may begin. These techniques are discussed later in this chapter.

BILATERAL CONTRACTION OF HIP FLEXOR MUSCLES

If the patient sits on the front portion of the chair and inclines the trunk backward until arrested by the back of the chair, a brief bilateral activation of the hip flexor muscles may be obtained. For greater range of motion, the patient makes a quarter turn on the chair toward the normal side or sits on a stool or bench without back support. The hip flexor muscles respond with a lengthening contraction when the trunk inclines backward and with a shortening contraction during the return movement. The abdominal muscles are activated as well. Most patients feel insecure at first and proper security measures must be taken, but few fail to accomplish this movement within small or moderately large range.

The flexor muscles of the hip may be employed either for balancing the trunk in an anteroposterior direction, or for flexing the thigh with respect to the trunk. Their bilateral trunk-balancing function is essentially an equilibrium reaction, evoked automatically to prevent a fall. Such function of the hip flexor muscles may be retained in patients with hemiplegia, while unilateral activation of the same muscles in flexing the thigh with respect to the trunk may fail to materialize. Trunk balance may thus be utilized as preparation for thigh flexion.

UNILATERAL CONTRACTION OF HIP FLEXOR MUSCLES

Immediately following a backward trunk inclination or while such inclination is still in progress, the patient makes an effort to flex the thigh with respect to the trunk. The timing of this attempt is critical, for it must be made before the tension in the hip flexor muscles, developed during trunk inclination, has subsided. Because muscles can produce more tension during isometric or lengthening contractions than during shortening contractions, the therapist assists in hip flexion just enough to lift the foot off the ground, then gives the command "Hold," or "Don't let your foot down on the floor." During this attempt the

patient sits on the front portion of the chair so that the trunk-thigh angle becomes obtuse.

ACTIVATING THE DORSIFLEXOR MUSCLES OF THE ANKLE

The close association that exists between the dorsiflexor muscles of the ankle and the hip flexor muscles in patients with hemiplegia was pointed out by Marie and Foix (1916), who classified the phenomenon as "coordination synkinesis" (see Abstract 17). In more recent years the linkage between these two groups of muscles has been referred to as "confusion movement" (Phelps, 1938; Egel, 1948). The latter term appears rather unsuitable since the two movements are component parts of a well-organized pattern.

By evoking the total flexor synergy of the lower limb while resisting its hip flexion component, a contraction of the dorsiflexor muscles of the ankle can almost always be brought about in patients with hemiplegia, provided some spasticity is present. The utilization of the synkinesis between the two muscle groups for training purposes is further discussed in Chapter 5.

UPPER LIMB TRAINING, STAGES 1 TO 3

Recovery Stages 1 to 3, as outlined in Chapter 2, cover the period following the onset of hemiplegia when the originally flaccid condition (Stage 1) comes to an end and spasticity begins to develop (Stage 2) then reaches its height (Stage 3). Simultaneously, the basic limb synergies gradually make their appearance, and the synergy influence on motor performance becomes marked, to the exclusion of other movement combinations.

Therapeutic procedures are instituted to promote voluntary control of the synergies by the patient and to assist him to use the synergies for purposeful activities. Reversal of movement direction in the paths of the two synergies is stressed as is painless range of motion at all joints. It is postulated that control, or partial control, of the basic movement synergies is a prerequisite for the development of more extensive motor control.

EVOKING ASSOCIATED REACTIONS

If the patient is unable to initiate voluntary movements and spasticity or potential spasticity is present, associated reactions may be utilized to evoke a background tension in flexor or extensor muscles in preparation for voluntary initiation of movement. The first associated reaction observed following the onset of hemiplegia usually occurs in the flexor muscles; extensor responses appear later.

When the associated response is weak, a tensing of the muscles without joint movement may be observed, but in most instances, if the patient's effort is strong, some joint movement may be observed, particularly if the eliciting stimulus is repeated. Semivoluntary movements may then materialize from an interaction of reflex and voluntary impulses, and the patient experiences the sensation and satisfaction that accompanies a voluntary muscular contraction. This is the main purpose of associated reactions in training procedures. The type of stimulus that elicits the desired muscular contraction also indicates to the therapist what type of resistance in other parts of the body is most effective to reinforce weak voluntary movements.

Figure 1-11 is an example of an unusually vivid, full-range associated flexion reaction in the left upper limb of a patient who could not initiate any voluntary movement in that limb. The complete reaction was first elicited several times. Then, when the arm had moved about half range, another therapist, standing on the patient's affected side, grasped the patient's forearm and gave the command, "Hold, don't let me pull your arm down." The patient was delighted to feel that he could resist. Later, a reversal from a lengthening to a shortening contraction was achieved, and before long the patient could perform the flexor synergy without resistance on the unaffected side.

Few patients demonstrate associated reactions in complete synergy range as did the patient referred to in the preceding paragraph. But as long as some associated reaction, however small, is evoked, it may be utilized for training purposes during the early recovery stages. Associated reactions serve no useful purpose in advanced training.

In the text that follows little or no mention is made of associated reactions, but it is understood that these reactions may be employed in conjunction with other facilitatory procedures.

FLEXION MOVEMENTS

These movements include passive, active guided and resisted movements in the path of the flexor synergy. Elbow flexion can usually be performed passively through the full range without pain, and it is usually one of the first components over which the patient gains voluntary control. But many problems arise when shoulder movements are first attempted. In the following discussion, therefore, shoulder problems are given special attention.

Shoulder Pain

A considerable number of patients with hemiplegia complain about shoulder pain when passive shoulder abduction to increase range of motion is attempted. However, nearly complete range of abduction without pain may be obtained with the patient's cooperation, i.e., if a combination of active and passive movements are utilized. Shoulder girdle movements—elevation, lowering, retraction, protraction—are first stressed, then in conjunction with these, painless glenohumeral movements of increased range become possible. Forceful shoulder movements with no regard to pain are ill-advised because they are of more hindrance than help.

Patients who have experienced severe pain from a forced passive range of motion procedure may become very apprehensive, even hostile. In such patients a protective mechanism, characterized by strong tension in the pectoralis major muscle and in other muscles surrounding the shoulder joint, may develop, which makes attempts at shoulder mobilization doubly difficult. These patients are kept on preliminary mobilization procedures as described earlier in this chapter until their fear of pain has been overcome. If such a patient is treated gently and realizes that, at his request, any movement causing pain will be stopped immediately, he may soon become cooperative, and his changed state of mind will be accompanied by a lessening of muscular tension about the shoulder joint.

Support of the Patient's Arm

A convenient way to support the patient's affected arm is illustrated in Figure 3-5. This manner of carrying the arm requires no change of grip when the physical therapist wishes to follow through with increasing range in the paths of the flexor and extensor synergies, including rotary movements of shoulder and forearm. The physical therapist's right hand is free to assist scapular rotation or for sensory stimulation.

Techniques for Painless Shoulder Movements

The procedure begins with shoulder elevation and lowering, first performed bilaterally, then unilaterally. The starting position of the arm for these movements is lower than the one seen in Figure 3-5A. The arm is supported with the elbow flexed.

If the patient is unable to elevate the shoulder girdle voluntarily, the movement is assisted by upward pressure on the elbow. Simultaneously, the physical therapist may use his free hand for percussion or cutaneous stimulation over the upper trapezius muscle. When the muscle responds, a lengthening contraction is first requested ("Don't let me push your shoulder down"), then elevation is repeated—if possible, against manual resistance ("Now pull your shoulder up toward your ear").

Shoulder elevation performed actively by the patient tends to evoke activity in all components of the flexor synergy, particularly if resistance is applied. It also has an inhibitory effect on components of the extensor synergy, notably on the pectoralis major muscle. This inhibition is utilized by the physical therapist to gently abduct the arm in small increments each time the patient repeats the movement. The rhythm of these repetitions is regulated by the therapist's voice as he directs the procedure: "Pull up, let go, pull up, let go," etc. The direction of these abduction movements is oblique, half way between forward and sideward; the strictly sideward direction is likely to cause pain and is avoided.

At one time or another during the elevation procedure the patient's attention is drawn to supination of the forearm. Note that alternate supination and pronation movements by the physical therapist has accompanied elevation and lowering all along. Because supination of the forearm and external rotation of the shoulder are mutually facilitatory (both belong to the flexor synergy), the two movements should be combined. External rotation of the shoulder, required for abduction beyond the horizontal, has thus been introduced painlessly, and the stage is set for further elevation of the arm. Head rotation toward the normal side usually contributes to relaxation of the pectoralis major muscle. The give-and-take method of increasing abduction range is continued (Fig. 3-5*B* and *C*).

After the arm has been carried well above the horizontal position and if no pain is present, the command "Reach overhead and straighten out your elbow" may be given. First, however, the patient must rotate the head toward the affected side to facilitate elbow extension and to allow him to observe the movement. The last portion of the procedure should only be requested of patients who have made sufficient progress.

It is equally effective to employ shoulder girdle *retraction* and its opposite movement, *protraction*, as a starting point for shoulder mobilization. Like shoulder elevation, shoulder retraction is comparatively easy for stroke patients to carry out. Elevation and retraction are both components of the flexor synergy, and both tend to produce tension in associated flexor muscles. Bilateral shoulder retraction ("pinching of the shoulders in the back," according to the patient) may be accentuated by cutaneous stimulation in the interscapular region. The therapist scratches or pinches the skin in a direction toward the vertebral column, which indicates to the patient where the movement should take place and which possibly facilitates the contraction of the required muscles.

The techniques described result in increased range of motion at the shoulder and also serve to organize and develop the flexor synergy. A small range movement in the opposite direction—that is, in the path of the extensor synergy—is performed between the patient's flexion efforts so that actually both synergies are being developed. As training progresses, special emphasis is given to the development of the extensor synergy. Eventually the two synergies are combined in a "roundabout" fashion, such as would result from the use of a shoulder wheel, with the additional movements of supination-external rotation and pronation-internal rotation incorporated in the guided movement.

Subluxation of the Shoulder Joint

Activation of the muscles surrounding the shoulder joint is needed, not only for the total functioning of the upper limb, but also to guard the shoulder joint from subluxation. Many muscles pass over the shoulder joint, and all of these combine to maintain the integrity of the joint, but there are good reasons to believe that the "cuff muscles"—the supraspinatus, infraspinatus, teres minor, and subscapularis—are particularly important for the prevention of glenohumeral separation.

Proper function of the deltoid muscle certainly is of great importance, but it would seem as if this muscle were less concerned with holding the humeral head close to the glenoid cavity than with glenohumeral movements as such. The author has seen several stroke patients who had good return of the deltoid muscle, yet glenohumeral separation was present. Whether or not the supraspinatus muscle remained inactive in these cases has not been determined satisfactorily, but its nonfunction appears likely. It has been shown by electromyography that under normal conditions the supraspinatus muscle, to a much greater extent than the deltoid muscle, increases its activity when a load is carried in the hand (Basmajian, 1966). This would indicate that the supraspinatus muscle is particularly important for the prevention of subluxation of the shoulder joint.

It is common practice to have patients with hemiplegia use an arm sling to prevent glenohumeral separation. Such a sling, if properly constructed and applied, aids in holding the humeral head in the socket but does not in any way stimulate the activity of muscles that are needed to protect the joint.

Reinforcement of Voluntary Abduction

A number of different approaches—several of these combined—may be employed to evoke and reinforce voluntary abduction efforts by the patient. The following are some general principles:

1. The entire flexor synergy is employed in order to take advantage of the facilita-

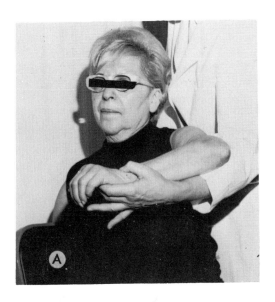

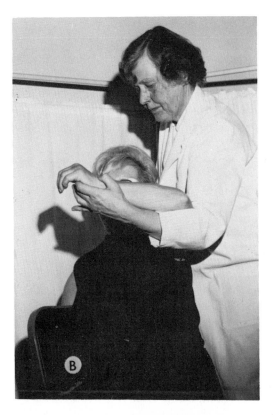

FIGURE 3-5. Support of affected arm for painless range of motion. Patient has a left-sided hemiparesis of 2 months' duration. *A.* The entire arm is supported, wrist extended. *B.* With the patient actively cooperating, increase of range at shoulder is obtained by small increments. A movement path halfway between shoulder flexion and shoulder abduction is recommended. *C.* Maximal painless range has been reached. The head has been rotated to the left to further decrease tension in the pectoralis major muscle (see text).

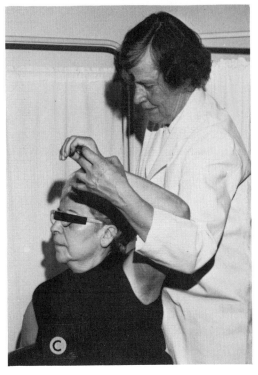

tory effect of the stronger components on the weaker ones.

2. Whenever feasible, resistance is applied.
3. The movements are guided so as to avoid pain.
4. The patient's effort is first requested for a flexor component over which he has at least partial control.
5. Local stimulation—proprioceptive and exteroceptive—of the poorly responding muscles is employed.
6. Facilitatory measures are repeated (such repetitions may have a cumulative effect).
7. Isometric and lengthening contractions are requested before shortening contractions.
8. The extensor synergy or some of its components are evoked momentarily for a succession of agonist-antagonist responses.

Head rotation toward the normal side may be used to decrease tension in the pectoralis major muscle, but this is not a universal rule. When position sense and passive motion sense are impaired or absent the patient often spontaneously turns his head toward the affected side because he needs visual guidance; this guidance may be of greater benefit to the patient than the facilitatory effect of the tonic neck reflex. (The possible advantage of an obliquely placed mirror to enable the patient to see his arm while the head is rotated toward the affected side has been investigated. In general, the mirror image of the arm appeared to confuse rather than to aid the patients investigated.)

It is difficult indeed to describe adequately when and how the above principles are applied. There has to be a continuous search for methods and combinations that bring results. Careful observation of each patient's reactions must always be a guideline, and experience gained in the treatment of one stroke patient can often be employed to advantage with other patients.

Use of Proximal Traction Response

During the spastic stage, weak voluntary contractions of components of the flexor synergy may be reinforced by a sudden stretch of or continuous traction on any one of the flexor muscles. Such stimulation results in reflex contraction not only of the stretched muscles but also of other muscles belonging to the flexor synergy (see Chapter 1). The flexor muscles of either shoulder, elbow, wrist, or digits may be subjected to this kind of stimulation, and when the response spreads to other flexor muscles, the command "Hold" (for isometric contraction) or "Pull" (for shortening contraction) is given. When the patient is seated, retraction of the shoulder girdle and hyperextension of the shoulder is part of the response so that a shortening of the entire limb, a "shortening synkinesis,"

results. The abduction component of the flexor synergy is not likely to appear during this procedure.

The proximal traction response is of limited value for training purposes and should be employed for selected patients only. For example, it may be desirable to evoke or reinforce a contraction of the flexor muscles of the elbow, or to reinforce the patient's grip in conjunction with a voluntary effort. However, wrist flexion is part of the proximal traction response, and wrist flexion is undesirable from a functional standpoint.

Following the use of the traction response, manipulations of forearm, wrist, and digits are undertaken for the purpose of transferring tension from the flexor to the extensor muscles. These manipulations are described later in this chapter.

EXTENSION MOVEMENTS

Bilateral Contraction of the Pectoralis Major Muscle

If the patient is unable to initiate any part of the extensor synergy, the pectoralis major muscle on the affected side can usually be activated by the utilization of a reaction comparable to Raimiste's phenomenon. Both the supine and the sitting positions lend themselves well to this procedure.

When this reaction is evoked in the sitting position, the therapist stands facing the patient and supports his arms in a horizontal position obliquely forward. Resistance is applied to the medial side of the normal arm just above the elbow as the patient is asked to adduct that arm horizontally. Firm resistance by the therapist brings the pectoralis major muscle into strong contraction, and after some latency a response is likely to appear also on the involved side. Voluntary bilateral contraction is now solicited by the command, "Don't let me pull your arms apart," followed by "Now, bring your arms toward each other again."

Reinforcement of Elbow Extension

Although tension in the pectoralis major muscle usually develops at an early date, elbow extension, a weak component of the extensor synergy, usually lags behind. During the period of synergy dominance, a contraction of the triceps muscles is only obtained in conjunction with that of the pectoralis major muscle, because shoulder and elbow components of the extensor synergy are firmly linked. Impulses of various origins may have to be set up if the patient is to succeed in extending the elbow complete range. Examples are as follows:

1. Head rotation toward the affected side. Aids in releasing tension in the flexor muscles of the elbow while simultaneously promoting a background tension in the triceps muscles.
2. Pronation of the forearm by the physical therapist or by the patient (who then uses his unaffected hand for that purpose) prior to the patient's effort to extend the elbow. The supinated position, seen in Figure 1-5, inhibits elbow extension.
3. Trunk rotation toward the normal side. The patient places his pronated forearm against the lateral side of the thigh on the normal side and pushes in a downward direction.
4. Vigorous back and forth stroking of the skin over the triceps muscles as the patient makes an effort to push, i.e., to extend the elbow.
5. Bilateral "rowing exercise" against resistance, an activity that takes advantage of the facilitatory effects of proprioceptive impulses originating on the normal side and in the trunk. The physical therapist, seated in front of the patient, guides the movement and offers resistance on the normal side and, as soon as possible, on the affected side as well. Trunk movements accompany the "rowing," as they would in a rowboat; series of repetitions are required. When the patient pushes, his forearms are pronated, and when he pulls they may be supinated if the therapist finds the right grip.

6. Unilateral resistance to a push movement in the path of the extensor synergy. May be applied with the therapist standing behind the patient or sitting in front of him. Resistance may be applied to the proximal portion of the patient's palm with a grip that also keeps the wrist extended, as in Figure 3-5, or with a grip over the patient's closed fist, as in Figure 3-6A. Such resistance gives direction to the patient's effort and often results in complete elbow extension even though the patient may be unable to accomplish this without resistance.

7. "Hold-after-positioning" technique. The affected arm is guided into nearly full range of the extensor synergy until the elbow is just short of full extension, as in Figure 3-6A. "Hold, don't let me push your arm back," is the command. A number of rapid, small-range, backward pushing movements by the therapist elicits a series of stretch reflexes in the triceps muscles which reinforce the patient's voluntary effort. The patient feels that he can offer resistance, and this is encouraging. A shortening contraction may then become possible.

8. Resistance by a sandbag placed on a low stool in front of the patient (Fig. 3-6B). An impression is first made in the sandbag to accommodate the patient's clenched fist. The patient leans forward and uses the normal hand to guide the affected hand to the sandbag. Once the fist has made contact with the sandbag the body weight is shifted onto the affected arm, which now has to function to support body weight as if it were the forelimb of a quadruped animal (compare Magnus, the positive supporting reaction, 1926, and Brain, the quadrupedal extensor reflex, 1927). The ex-

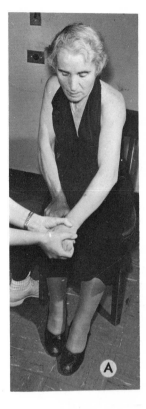
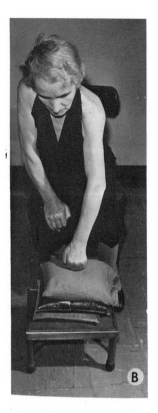

FIGURE 3-6. Eliciting and reinforcing elbow extension in a 58-year-old patient with left-sided hemiparesis, 10 months after a cerebral vascular accident. *A.* "Hold-after-positioning" technique (see text). *B.* Activation and reinforcement of elbow extensor muscles by weight shift over the affected upper limb. Body posture resembles that of a quadruped animal (see text). (*B* from Brunnstrom, S. Methods used to elicit, reinforce, and coordinate muscular response in adult patients with hemiplegia. In *Correlation of Physiology with Therapeutic Exercise, APTA-OVR Institute Papers.* New York, American Physical Therapy Association, 1956, p. 100.)

tensor muscles of the elbow seldom fail to respond to this challenge.

9. Use of the supine position. If at an early date poor results are obtained with the patient seated, the supine position may be chosen for training. Because of labyrinthine influence (Magnus and de Kleijn 1912), this position markedly favors extension. The facilitatory influence of the supine posi-

tion on elbow extension is demonstrated by the patient in Figure 2-1*B–D*.

WITHDRAWAL OF THERAPIST'S ASSISTANCE

So far, the physical therapist has utilized certain techniques to aid the patient to perform movements in the path of the basic limb synergies. He has guided, assisted, and resisted the movement synergies and their individual components, has introduced reversal of movement direction, and has step by step outlined and directed the procedures. Assistance must now gradually be withdrawn so that the patient becomes independent of the therapist for basic synergy movements.

PRACTICAL USE OF THE BASIC LIMB SYNERGIES

Movement therapy becomes more meaningful if the patient can utilize whatever control he has gained from the above procedures for functional activities. Even though at this time the control of the affected arm is limited, it may be used in many ways. Without it, the patient would have to function as a one-armed individual.

During the synergy stages, the affected arm serves as an aid to the normal arm, which must be relied on for all major activities, skilled and unskilled. Advantage may be taken of the patient's control of flexor as well as extensor components, and of the entire synergies when these are under control.

The extensor synergy may be used as follows:

1. To stabilize an object on the table while the unaffected hand opens an envelope or writes a letter. Such stabilization is also useful for many household activities.
2. To stabilize an object between the affected arm and the body. A jar may be held steady while the unaffected hand unscrews its top; a handbag or

a newspaper may be held under the arm while the unaffected hand opens a door; etc.

3. To push the affected arm through a sleeve while the normal hand holds the garment in such a position that the movement may follow the path of the extensor synergy. (First, however, the forearm must be pronated, for if it remains supinated or semisupinated, elbow extension is inhibited.)

The flexor synergy or its components may be utilized for many activities:

1. To carry a coat over the forearm, elbow flexed, provided the elbow flexor muscles are sufficiently strong.
2. To carry a briefcase or handbag after the handles have been placed in the hand. The grip of the affected hand, however, can seldom be relied upon for any length of time, because the grip may loosen if the patient's attention does not remain focused on hand closure.
3. To hold a small object in the hand, such as a toothbrush, while the normal hand squeezes dental cream on the brush; to hold a matchbook between the thumb and the index finger while striking a match.

Two-handed pulling and pushing activities, such as handling a broom, carpet sweeper, or vacuum cleaner, or dusting a table, may be performed, but for these activities the normal hand may have to stabilize the affected one. Only strongly motivated patients will use these movements because the affected hand may be of more hindrance than help. Under the supervision of a therapist, however, these activities become therapeutic procedures that most patients are willing to try.

UPPER LIMB TRAINING, STAGES 4 AND 5

Spasticity is now on the decline, and synergy dominance over motor acts is waning. The effectiveness of voluntary effort is on the increase, which enables the patient to learn a number of comparatively easy movement combinations that deviate from the basic synergies (Stage 4), then to proceed to more difficult combinations (Stage 5). However, control of individual joint movements is not yet to be expected. Training procedures aim at modifying the available motor responses and reinforcing the willed impulses to overcome the still existing, although diminishing, linkage between synergy components.

INTRODUCING VARIATIONS IN MOVEMENT DIRECTIONS

It is not necessary to wait for the completion of full range of motion of all components of the two basic synergies before variations are attempted. However, a certain level of control of the synergies must have been reached. The patient must have learned to perform "pull" and "push" movements, for his ability to do so constitutes the basis for the development of movements that deviate from the paths of the synergies.

At this stage the patient does not know how to initiate a movement that carries no resemblance to either of the synergies. Many functional activities, however, have a flexor or extensor character, and these are the ones that are tackled at this time. An attempt is made to modify the patient's voluntary muscular responses—i.e., the flexor and the extensor synergies—to enable him to perform a variety of related movements and functional activities.

Flexor Activities

If the path of the flexor synergy is followed and the shoulder components are strong, the hand arrives at positions such as those seen in Figures 1-1 and 3-7A. In order that the hand may reach the mouth or contact various points on the trunk and head, the shoulder components (abduction

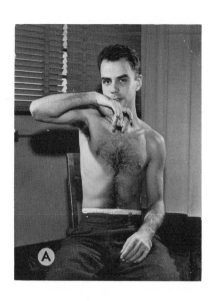 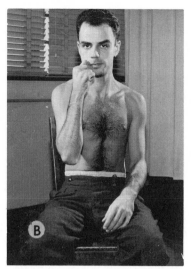 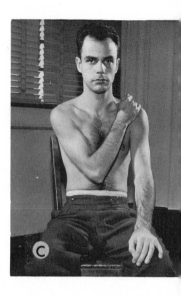

and external rotation) must be modified or be replaced by an extensor component (pectoralis major muscle). The patient in Figure 3-7 illustrates such modification of the flexor synergy. While learning the new combination, he had to perform the hand-to-mouth and hand-to-opposite-shoulder movements in two stages. First, he inhibited abduction by pressing the elbow firmly against the side of the body; second, he flexed the elbow and the hand was directed to the designated spot. After some practice, two separate movements were no longer necessary, although the patient had to concentrate on the task to prevent the shoulder from abducting.

Patients with weak shoulder components (Figs. 1-5 and 1-6) have a somewhat different problem. They fail to reach the mouth because of retraction of the arm at the shoulder and because of weak elbow flexors. The flexor muscles of the elbow must then be strengthened by applying facilitatory techniques, such as direct muscle stimulation (proprioceptive or cutaneous), "hold-after-positioning" technique, etc.

The movements listed below are given as examples of activities which may be practiced to promote a transition between Stages 3 and 4. These activities are all derived from the flexor synergy and based

FIGURE 3-7. A 23-year-old patient with right-sided hemiparesis of traumatic origin, 5 years after injury. _A._ When patient was asked to bring the hand to the mouth, the arm abducted and the head turned to meet the hand. _B._ Abduction is inhibited by pressing the elbow firmly against the side of the body while flexing the elbow. _C._ "Hand-to-opposite shoulder" requires inhibition of abduction and activation of the pectoralis major muscle during elbow flexion.

on the patient's ability to initiate elbow flexion. The desired movement paths are first demonstrated to the patient by repeated passive movements which cause the patient's hand to touch a designated spot on the head or on the trunk, or to slide over a specific body area. The sensory impulses thus set up are believed to facilitate the voluntary movement to be attempted; they appear to give direction to the patient's effort. The movements are:

1. Hand to chin (Fig. 3-7*B*)
2. Hand to ear, to touch the ear first on the affected then on the unaffected side; head rotation is allowed
3. Hand to touch opposite elbow
4. Hand to opposite shoulder (Fig. 3-7*C*)
5. Hand to forehead
6. Hand to top of head
7. Hand to back part of head
8. Stroking movements

A. Starting on the forehead, stroking over the top of the head to the back part of the head
B. Starting with both hands in the lap, the affected hand performs a stroking movement over the dorsum of the forearm on the normal side and follows the arm up toward the shoulder or beyond the shoulder toward the neck

For these stroking movements it would be desirable to have the patient use the palm of his hand, but if this is not possible because of tension in the finger flexor muscles, stroking is carried out with closed fist.

The activities listed above require mainly a grading of intensity of various flexor components, an emphasis on one component or the other, not a completely new association of muscles. The only extensor component to be recruited for some of the movements is the pectoralis major muscle. The association of this muscle with flexor components is not very difficult to achieve because the muscle usually possesses a background tension at an early date. In fact, shoulder adduction and elbow flexion often combine spontaneously to produce the "typical arm posture" in hemiplegia, as seen in Figure 1-10. Thus, no influences that strongly antagonize each other are introduced in the above activities.

As soon as feasible, functional activities are stressed. Successful completion of such activities gives a boost to the patient's motivation; establishing a purpose for a movement aids in developing the required coordination; and contact with a body part where sensation is intact no doubt is instrumental in guiding the hand to its destination. A piece of bread is placed in the patient's hand and he is encouraged to bring it to his mouth; he is given a comb in his affected hand to try to comb his hair; a washcloth may be placed in his hand so that he can learn to wash the arm on the opposite side and to reach the axilla; and so on.

Extensor Activities

When the patient is seated, the path of the extensor synergy brings the hand to a position just above the knee on the affected side, as in Figure 1-2*B*, often to a more adducted position between the two knees. The pectoralis major muscle, which becomes strongly activated whenever elbow extension is willed, is responsible for the movement direction of the extensor synergy. A modification in the intensity of contraction of this muscle, particularly of its lower portion, is required for extension movements in a forward direction, as in reaching out for an object in front of the body. For more lateral extensor movements the pectoralis major muscle must become disassociated from the triceps muscles. When such disassociation is complete, the basic limb synergies no longer dominate the patient's motor acts.

The breaking up of the linkage between the triceps and the pectoralis major muscles requires a step-by-step modification of the voluntarily performed extensor synergy. For this purpose, the physical therapist repeatedly resists extension movements and guides them into slightly different directions. The patient's primary responsibility is to push, which he has already learned to do. The guided resisted movements begin in a forward-downward direction and gradually reach the horizontal plane, then proceed in a more lateral direction; they are also guided into downward and backward directions. The latter movements are important because they prepare for the activation of a number of posterior muscles needed to bring the hand behind the body. A strictly side horizontal extensor movement is not attempted; it is too difficult at this time. If range of motion at shoulder is painless and free, guided oblique extensor movements in an upward direction may also begin.

Stroking movements with contact on body parts may now be extended to all areas of the thighs and may continue over the knees and as far down on the legs as the patient can conveniently reach. These movements require modification of the extensor synergy, reversal of movement directions, and adjustment of the forearm with respect to pronation and supination. Guidance by the physical therapist is essential at first because coordination develops only gradually.

The following are examples of functional activities that require flexor and extensor movements and that are suitable at this time: Pushing the affected arm through a coat sleeve; pushing away an object on a table; opening and closing a drawer; using a sanding or polishing block. Many activities consisting of alternate pulling and pushing are best started bilaterally. If the patient has fair control of the lower limb, activities such as walking around the room and dusting furniture, using a push-broom, a carpet sweeper, or a vacuum cleaner may be introduced.

It was pointed out in Chapter 2 that a progression from synergy dominance to decrease of such dominance and eventually to independence of the synergies is the sequence employed by nature in restoring motor function. In planning neuromuscular therapy, this sequence must be followed. If the patient is to progress from Stage 3 to Stages 4 and 5, movement combinations must be introduced which deviate from the paths of the basic limb synergies. For this purpose, a breaking up of the strong linkage that exists between certain components of each of the basic synergies is required; in addition, muscle groups that do not belong to either synergy must begin to function.

Examples of three comparatively easy motor achievements chosen to represent Stage 4 and three more difficult ones to represent Stage 5, together with a discussion of training techniques, follow.

ARM TO REAR OF BODY (Stage 4)

Neither the flexor synergy nor the extensor synergy provides muscular combinations required for bringing the entire arm behind the body, as needed for washing the back portion of the body, adjusting clothing, and reaching into a back pocket. Certain muscles in the back must be induced to function, such as the latissimus dorsi, the teres major, and the rhomboids. The pectoralis major muscle must become disassociated from elbow extension, and it may be assumed that the participation of the subscapularis muscle as an internal rotator of the shoulder is also required.

Placing the arm behind the body is not as difficult a movement as it may seem at first. Although it appears to bear no resemblance to either of the two basic limb synergies, the movement may evolve from these synergies as follows.

Starting with the Flexor Synergy

The patient elevates the shoulder girdle, hyperextends and slightly abducts the shoulder, and flexes the elbow, while allowing the forearm to hang in a more or less vertical position with the dorsum of the hand touching the lateral part of the hip. The woman in Figure 3-8A has accomplished this movement and has brought the hand slightly toward the rear. From this point on, the extensor synergy takes over and the hand is pushed obliquely downward across the sacrum toward the opposite side, as in Figure 3-8B. Small pulling and pushing movements are now performed, causing the dorsum of the hand to rub up and down over the skin in the back. For reinforcement of muscular contraction and to emphasize surface stimulation, these movements, particularly the pushing part, may be resisted by the physical therapist.

If the patient finds it difficult to move the hand beyond the lateral position, the physical therapist assists that portion of the movement by internally rotating the shoulder. During the pushing movement, a strong contraction of the pectoralis major muscle may be expected, but with repetition this contraction gradually becomes less and the posterior muscles begin to function. It may be assumed that impulses originating from the area of the trunk, which is stimulated, together with afferent impulses from joints, muscles, and skin of the affected upper limb, are instrumental in shunting impulses into the desired efferent pathways. Guidance by the physical therapist and contact with the patient's hand on the trunk may be required for some time before the patient succeeds to bring the arm backward as a free movement.

Starting with the Extensor Synergy

The patient performs successive pushing movements in forward, obliquely sideward, downward, and backward directions. These movements are guided and resisted by the physical therapist, and when the arm has arrived behind the body the dorsum of the patient's hand is rubbed over the sacral region, as described above.

Rhythmic, alternate, forward and backward extension movements guided by the physical therapist are introduced next.

Between each extension movement, the arm passes through a flexion phase, as in Figure 3-8A. Reversal of movement directions, not only from flexion to extension, but also from extension forward to extension backward, is thus accomplished. The rhythm of the movements may be regulated by the physical therapist's words: "Pull, reach forward; pull, reach back." Eventually, these movements are performed without the patient's hand making contact with the body.

Starting with Trunk Rotation, Standing Erect

If balance is satisfactory, the patient stands erect with the feet a few inches

FIGURE 3-8. Same patient as in Figure 3-5. The synergies of flexion and extension are modified to bring the hand behind the body. *A.* Components of the flexor synergy bring the hand to the lateral side of the hip. *B.* The extensor synergy, resisted by the physical therapist, completes the movement (see text).

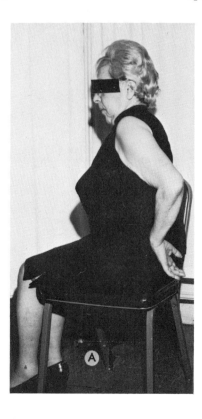
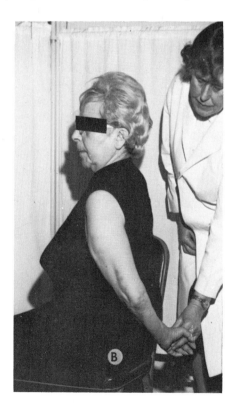

apart and the arms hanging as relaxed as possible at the sides of the body. Trunk rotation movements, gradually increasing in range, are begun, and the patient is told to let the arms "flop around" without trying to control them. Trunk rotation is not confined to a movement between chest and pelvis—the hips are allowed to participate. The trunk movements are performed rhythmically, and they set the arms in motion so that the arms are wrapped around the body first toward one side, then toward the other. If during this movement guidance of the arms is necessary, the physical therapist stands behind the patient and assists the arm movements, taking care not to throw him off balance. During trunk rotation to the left, the aim for the right hand is to "slap" the region of the greater trochanter on the left side, while the left arm swings to the rear so that the dorsum of the hand hits the back side of the body. The terms *slap* and *hit* have been used to indicate that the contact with the body is a sudden and audible one, the rhythm of which may be emphasized by a repetitious "touch, touch, touch," uttered by the physical therapist.

ARM-RAISING FORWARD TO HORIZONTAL POSITION (Stage 4)

Arm-raising forward with the elbow extended, when performed in a normal manner, is accomplished by the action of many muscles—those which produce scapulothoracic movements and those which control the glenohumeral and the elbow joints. Neither the flexor synergy nor the extensor synergy provides the exact muscular combinations required for this movement.

When flexor synergy influence cannot be overcome and the patient attempts to raise the arm forward, the arm tends to move into partial abduction, the elbow cannot be kept extended, and often the forearm remains partially supinated. If the patient begins with the total extensor synergy, the elbow extends but elevation of the arm is hindered, because of the contraction of the pectoralis major muscle, particularly its lower portion.

To facilitate the accomplishment of the desired movement, the patient makes an active effort while the physical therapist guides the movement and gives local stimulation where needed. If the patient succeeds in raising the arm to a near horizontal position but the elbow is incompletely extended, stroking or rubbing the skin over the triceps muscles reinforces the patient's effort to extend the elbow. Simultaneously, full forearm pronation must be present. When little or no elevation of the arm by the patient succeeds, manipulations or percussion over the anterior and middle portion of the deltoid muscle while the arm is passively elevated, followed by the "Hold" command, may be tried. In some patients the flexor synergy is first evoked for the purpose of relaxing the pectoralis major muscle and activating the deltoid muscle; then the arm is brought forward and the elbow extended without allowing the patient to make a strong effort.

When a "hold after positioning" is successful, small up-and-down movements of the arm, elbow extended, are begun, then range is increased until the entire movement of elevation and lowering is performed.

PRONATION-SUPINATION OF FOREARMS, ELBOWS FLEXED (Stage 4)

This is one of the first more or less isolated joint movements to be acquired when synergy influence is declining. Prior to such time, pronation only succeeds in combination with elbow extension and supination only in combination with elbow extension and supination only in combination with elbow flexion.

The patient is seated, elbows flexed, and both forearms are supported in the lap or resting on a pillow placed in the lap. The elbows are raised off the lap and the patient is instructed to keep the elbows in contact with the trunk while turning the palms up and down. A bilateral performance is preferred because it aids in preventing side movements of the trunk and because the performance on the two sides can then be compared (Fig. 2-3).

The flexed position of the elbow favors supination, and this movement may be expected to succeed, unless marked spasticity of the pronator muscles is present. After the forearm on the affected side has been fully supinated, the patient may be unable to initiate pronation. However, by moving the elbow away from the trunk and employing abduction-internal rotation of the shoulder, the forearm will fall into pronation by its own weight. This manner of pronating the forearm must not be confused with true pronation. Hence, when pronation-supination is given as a test, maintaining the elbows in contact with the trunk is mandatory.

If the patient is unable to initiate pronation with the elbow flexed, the following training method may be employed. The physical therapist pronates the patient's forearm the full range, while partially extending the elbow. In this position the patient is asked to push forward, a movement which is prevented by resistance. The command, "Don't let me turn your palm up," is given. Because the pronator muscles have become tensed as a component part of the extensor synergy, the patient may be expected to use these muscles to resist supination, although his attention has been switched from elbow extension to holding the forearm pronated. If the patient can resist supination, i.e., use the pronators in an isometric or a lengthening contraction, the movement direction is reversed: "Now turn your palm down again." By repeating the procedure while gradually increasing elbow flexion, the original position in which pronation was requested is approached. When resistance can be eliminated and the patient is able to pronate and supinate the forearm while

keeping the elbow close to the trunk, the goal has been reached.

The picture is somewhat different if a pronator contracture is present and if the pronator muscles are markedly spastic, a condition that is frequently encountered if the hemiparesis is of long standing. Some patients develop spasticity in the pronator muscles in a surprisingly short period of time. Spasticity in the pronator muscles, however, does not necessarily mean that the patient has the ability to initiate pronation voluntarily. Therefore, also under these circumstances, pronation-supination movements must be learned. In those cases, resistance to supination must also be emphasized for the purpose of lessening pronator tension and for increasing range of supination. When the supinator component of the flexor synergy is weak, not only must the ability to initiate the two movements be acquired, but strength in supination must be developed.

ARM-RAISING TO SIDE-HORIZONTAL POSITION (Stage 5)

The difficulty that a patient with hemiplegia experiences at an early recovery stage when attempting to elevate the arm to a side-horizontal position with the elbow extended is well illustrated in Figure 2-4A. This patient made an effort to perform the desired movement by starting with the flexor synergy over which she had good control, but with the shoulder abducted and externally rotated and the forearm supinated she was unable to inhibit the flexor muscles of the elbow, and the elbow remained flexed.

If a patient in such an early stage attempts to raise the arm laterally to a horizontal position, starting with the arm hanging at the side of the body, he may accomplish some abduction of the arm, but the elbow tends to flex because of the strong linkage that exists between the flexor muscles of the elbow and the abductor muscles of the shoulder. If the movement is to be performed correctly, two components of the extensor synergy (extension of the elbow and pronation of the forearm) must associate with two components of the flexor synergy (shoulder girdle retraction and shoulder abduction). Such mixing of synergy components is not easy for patients with hemiplegia because two competing influences are present and the patient's voluntary effort is insufficient to harmonize muscle action. A perfect performance of this movement, as seen in Figure 2-4B, is a sign that synergy influence is minimal or has altogether vanished.

ARM-RAISING OVERHEAD (Stage 5)

It is well known that a patient with an isolated paralysis of the serratus anterior muscle resulting from a peripheral nerve lesion is unable to raise the arm overhead; in fact, such a patient does not succeed in raising the arm above the horizontal position. In patients with hemiplegia, the flexor synergy, when complete, causes the arm to abduct 90 degrees but not beyond this point. One may therefore suspect that the serratus anterior muscle lies idle, particularly when it can be ascertained by inspection and palpation that the trapezius and the deltoid muscles contract strongly, as was the case in the patient in Figure 1-1B. This assumption is further borne out by the observation that in this stage patients with hemiplegia often display a marked winging of the scapula when an attempt is made to raise the arm forward and overhead (Fig. 3-9A). The position of the scapula seen in Figure 3-9A shows a striking resemblance to that seen in patients with lesions of the long thoracic nerve.

If in the sitting or standing position a patient is to succeed in raising the affected arm overhead to a vertical or near vertical position, painless range of motion at the shoulder must be present; the pectoralis major muscle must allow elongation without offering resistance; and the serratus anterior muscle as well as the glenohumeral muscles must function satisfactorily.

Techniques employed for achieving painless range of motion at the shoulder, for relaxing the pectoralis major muscle, and for evoking responses in the glenohumeral muscles have already been discussed. The approach suggested to facilitate the contraction of the serratus anterior muscle will be dealt with presently. For these methods to be potentially successful, a certain amount of control of muscles belonging to the two basic limb synergies is a prerequisite. The techniques cannot be applied to a patient whose upper limb is essentially flaccid.

Passive mobilization of the scapula previously described may be repeated here before active participation by the patient is requested. For such mobilization the therapist grasps around the medial border of the scapula to aid its forward sliding and its upward rotary movement on the rib cage as the arm is being elevated.

The training procedures to be described are first rehearsed on the unaffected side to ascertain that the patient fully understands what is expected of him and so that he experiences the accompanying sensations.

Stimulation of the serratus anterior muscle may begin with the patient's arm supported in a forward-horizontal position.

FIGURE 3-9. Techniques used to activate the serratus anterior muscle. The patient, age 48, has a right-sided hemiparesis of 11 months' standing. *A.* Maximal arm elevation prior to manipulations. The winging of the scapula suggests a nonfunctioning serratus anterior muscle. *B.* The arm has been positioned overhead. The physical therapist pushes the arm in a downward direction, using small jerky movements. *C.* Resistance is applied to arm-to-ear movement (see text). *D.* Following manipulations and positioning of arm, the patient maintains the arm well above the horizontal position. (*A* to *D* from Brunnstrom, S. Methods used to elicit, reinforce, and coordinate muscular response in adult patients with hemiplegia. In *Correlation of Physiology with Therapeutic Exercise, APTA-OVR Institute Papers.* New York, American Physical Therapy Association, 1956, p. 100.)

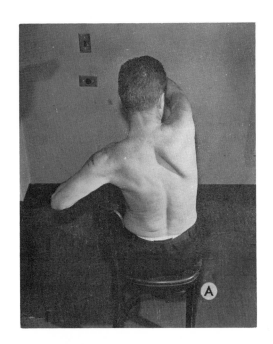

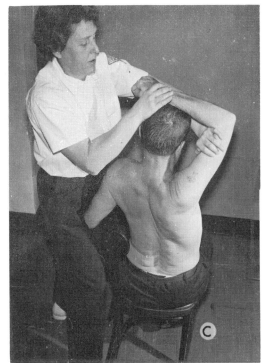

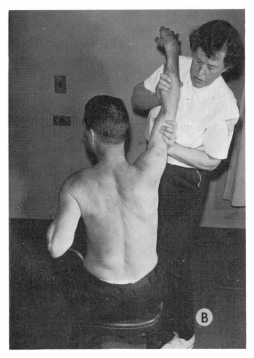

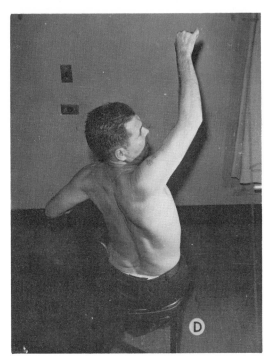

After requesting him to reach forward—a movement that is assisted—the therapist briskly pushes the arm backward in an attempt to evoke a stretch reflex in the serratus anterior muscle. Simultaneously, he gives the command, "Don't let me push your arm back." The patient's attempt to comply may result in a strong contraction of the pectoralis major muscle, but this will not bring the desired result. To avoid the contraction of the latter muscle, the arm must be brought into a more lateral position and the stimulation repeated.

Next the patient's arm is raised obliquely upward, eventually to an almost vertical position, as seen in Figure 3-9B. With the grip shown in the illustration, a number of rapidly repeated downward pushing movements are executed, and the physical therapist calls out, "Don't let me push your arm down," followed by "Reach for the sky." If an active upward reach does not materialize, the procedure is repeated. In the case of the patient illustrated, the serratus anterior muscle "caught on" after several repetitions, and when this happened the upward reach was reinforced by resistance.

As an alternative to the above procedure, the "arm-to-ear" movement illustrated in Figured 3-9C is recommended. When the sequence begins, the arm is supported, as in Figure 3-5A. The patient is told to move the arm in front of the body and reach toward the opposite shoulder; this movement is resisted. With each repetition the arm is raised to a somewhat higher position until the patient's hand is above his head, as in Figure 3-9C.

The patient's active effort is requested throughout this series of motions, and his task is simple to "pull over," a movement over which he has good control from the beginning. As the arm is being passively raised by small increments, the anterior portion, then also the middle portion, of the deltoid muscle become active. The final movement when the arm touches the ear requires full range in upward rotation of the scapula, and if the movement is resisted strongly, a spreading of efferent impulses to the serratus anterior muscle may be anticipated.

After the serratus anterior muscle has responded to one or both of the above manipulations, the patient must learn to maintain the arm elevated by himself. The arm is positioned overhead, and when response is felt the command "Hold" is given and the therapist takes his hands off so that the patient is on his own. Partial success is demonstrated by the man in Figure 3-9D: complete success is shown in Figure 2-5C, by a patient who had reached Stage 6. An emphatic "Don't let your arm fall down," or "Don't you *dare* let your arm fall down," seems further to reinforce the patient's voluntary effort. The last command must not be given unless the therapist is reasonably sure that the patient has the ability to comply. Experience with this technique is required before a prediction can be made concerning the patient's ability to "obey" the command.

TURNING PALMS UP AND DOWN, ELBOWS EXTENDED (Stage 5)

Of the three movements chosen to represent Stage 5, this has proven the most difficult one. Any remaining synergy influence, however slight, becomes evident during this movement.

In the sitting (or standing) position, the patient raises the arm to a side-horizontal position, elbow extended and forearm pronated. This movement combines two components of the flexor synergy with two components of the extensor synergy. When the palms are turned up, two more flexor components (supination of forearm and external rotation at shoulder) are added. This automatically draws in elbow flexion, because the only remaining antagonistic component, elbow extension, does not have a chance against the strong influence of four flexor components. The patient's voluntary effort to maintain the elbow extended only moderates the amount of elbow flexion; it does not suffice to suppress it. It is interesting to observe a patient in this stage who practices the palm-turning movements: each time the palm is turned up, the elbow flexes; when the palm is turned down, the elbow extends. With much concentration, such a patient may succeed in maintaining the elbow nearly extended, but the movements are then slow and strained and characterized by co-contraction of antagonistic muscles.

Performing the above movements with the arm in a forward-horizontal position is not much easier; also in this position the elbow tends to flex when the palm faces upward. Bilateral performance is preferred during practice to enable the patient to observe both hands in action. The difficulty become more marked if speed is increased.

The above movements are important from a testing standpoint, as they indicate where the patient stands with respect to recovery of the central nervous system. But from a functional standpoint they are rather unimportant. At this time, training procedures should emphasize useful activities involving pronation-supination movements in various arm positions and, in general, the application of the patient's existing controls to the tasks at hand. Activities that require the "mixing" of synergy components commensurable with the patient's recovery status are chosen. The patient's pre-stroke skills and interests should be cultivated rather than the learning of new skills. In most activities, the affected hand, whether the dominant or nondominant, remains a "helping hand," because throughout Stage 5 it is likely to retain a certain awkwardness. Two-handed activities are challenging to the patient, while the practice of one-handed skills using the affected hand may become frustrating—the normal hand can do the job much better and much faster.

In Stage 5, *relatively* isolated joint movements may become possible, such as flexion-extension of the elbow with the forearm pronated; forward-backward movements of the arms at the shoulder with the arms pendant; and rotary movements of the shoulder in certain arm positions. If a relatively isolated joint movement is to be attempted, the patient should first demonstrate his ability on the normal side. Functional activities seldom, if ever, require fully isolated movements of joints.

UPPER LIMB TRAINING, STAGE 6

In the sixth recovery stage, synergy influence has vanished or at least cannot easily be demonstrated. Movement combinations, including those listed for Stage 5, are under control and easily accomplished. Resistance to passive movements is no longer felt—that is, spasticity has disappeared. Individual joint movements of shoulder, elbow, forearm, and wrist are well performed in a normal or near normal fashion. Recovery of the hand, however, usually lags behind the rest of the limb. The patient may be able to use advanced prehension types, but when applying these to skilled activities the hand feels awkward. Therefore, the patient continues to favor it and uses it mainly as a secondary hand.

WHO REACHES STAGE 6?

Only those patients who make comparatively rapid recovery following a stroke may be expected to arrive at this advanced recovery stage. The woman patient who was followed over a period of 6 months and whose sequence of recovery is illustrated in Figures 2-4 to 2-6, 2-9 to 2-12, and 3-16 to 3-18 and 3-20 is an example. Seven weeks following a cerebral vascular accident she had fulfilled the requirements for Stage 4 and was entering Stage 5. Thereafter, she progressed through Stage 5 to Stage 6. Six months after the onset of hemiplegia the control of the limb as a whole was practically normal, but the hand remained awkward. Skilled hand activities are the "least automatic" and the "most voluntary" human motions (Jackson,

1884) and seldom recover completely after a stroke.

TRAINING ASPECTS

Specific training techniques cannot very well be outlined for Stage 6, because the approach must vary from patient to patient. The selection of tasks must be geared to overcome the specific difficulties encountered, and if these difficulties cannot be overcome, a compromise must be made. Much depends upon the patient's own motivation, determination, and persistence. The therapist's role is mainly to encourage and advise and to maintain a personal interest in the patient's welfare.

HAND TRAINING

The training techniques discussed above concerned the upper limb as a whole without emphasizing the problems of the hand. This does not mean that the hand should be neglected as the recovery proceeds from stage to stage. On the contrary, hand training commensurable with the recovery status of the patient is undertaken in all stages. Because control of the hand presents very specific problems and requires specific techniques, it was found more convenient to deal with it in a separate section.

The effectiveness of the hand as a tool is importantly related to the function of the entire upper limb. This must be kept continuously in mind as hand training proceeds. The first goal set for the hand, however, is the acquisition of mass grasp and mass release of objects. When this goal has been reached the patient is ready to learn more refined prehension activities.

GRASP ELICITED BY PROXIMAL TRACTION RESPONSE

If the patient is unable to initiate fist closure on a voluntary basis but has some control of the proximal components of the flexor synergy, resistance to the available joint movements may result in reflex activation of the muscles that flex the digits; wrist flexion (which is undesirable) is usually evoked simultaneously. This reaction, the *proximal traction response,* is likely to be present shortly after spasticity has developed (see Chapter 1). When this response is evoked for training purposes, the therapist maintains the wrist extended and the patient is told to squeeze. The interaction between reflex and voluntary impulses may result in partial fist closure even when the reflex alone or voluntary effort alone does not produce visible results. Once the patient has experienced the feeling that accompanies the initiation of finger flexion, he may soon be able to increase the range of fist closure and strengthen the grip, but wrist extension must be substituted for wrist flexion.

WRIST FIXATION FOR GRASP

Normally, a strong linkage exists between the muscles that stabilize the wrist in extension and those that flex the fingers. This linkage is commonly disturbed following a cerebral vascular accident and must be reestablished to render grasp effective.

Synergy Influence on Wrist Muscles

The flexor synergy, whether voluntarily performed or evoked as an associated reaction, is usually accompanied by wrist flexion (Figs. 1-5, 1-6, 1-7, 1-14), but wrist extension may also be observed (Figs. 1-8, 1-12). A wrist drop may persist for a considerable time whenever the elbow flexes, even though the patient makes good progress in other respects (Fig. 2-9B and C).

The extensor synergy is mostly accompanied by fixation of the wrist in extension, and this is true whether the synergy is evoked as an associated reaction (Fig. 1-2A), performed semivoluntarily (Fig. 1-2B), or carried out altogether voluntarily

(Fig. 2-9*A*). Although exceptions occur, there are good reasons for the statement that, fundamentally, wrist extension is a component part of the extensor synergy. Patients often acquire the ability to stabilize the wrist in extension when the elbow is extended long before such stabilization is possible when the elbow flexes. The patient shown in Figures 2-9*A* and 2-9*D* exemplifies the rule.

Wrist Positioning

When a wrist-drop is present, the therapist supports the patient's wrist in extension, as in Figure 3-5, whenever he moves the arm passively. If during active extension movements resistance is applied to the proximal portion of the patient's palm or to his closed fist, such resistance also serves to maintain the wrist dorsiflexed. Patients are also shown how to position the wrist in dorsiflexion by using the normal hand and when pushing against an object with closed fist (Fig. 3-6*B*). Positioning the wrist is considered important as it evokes afferent impulses that may favorably influence the motor responses.

Percussion of Wrist Extensor Muscles

To facilitate wrist fixation for grasp, the wrist is positioned as described, and the arm, elbow extended, is supported by the physical therapist. Stretch reflexes are evoked by percussion over the proximal portions of the wrist extensor muscles; simultaneously, the command "squeeze" is given in an attempt to synchronize the contraction of wrist extensor and finger flexor muscles. A stretch reflex of the extensor carpi radialis longus muscle is easily evoked, but the other two wrist extensor muscles will also respond if percussion is given over their muscle bellies. The "Squeeze" and "Stop squeezing" commands are alternated. At the proper time, while the patient is squeezing, the wrist support is withdrawn and the command

"Hold" is given, which implies that the patient must maintain the wrist extended while continuing to flex the fingers. If necessary, rapidly repeated percussion movements continue while the patient makes an effort to hold the position.

Once the desired synchronization of muscles has been achieved, firm fist closure is alternated with a "wrist-drop" (relaxation of wrist extensor and finger flexor muscles). On the "Stop squeezing" command the arm is carried backward so that the elbow flexes; the arm is again carried forward as the command "Squeeze" is given, because elbow extension has a favorable effect on wrist extension and elbow flexion promotes relaxation of the wrist extensor muscles.

Wrist Stabilization for Grasp, Elbow Flexed

When wrist stabilization for grasp has been well established with the elbow extended, a modification process begins to enable the patient to retain the newly acquired muscular association with the elbow in flexion as well as in extension. The entire process of positioning, percussion, fist closure, and "hold" by the patient is repeated with the elbow slightly flexed, taking care that the forearm is fully pronated. Elbow flexion is then gradually increased until the affected hand reaches the chin. The woman in Figure 1-7 was exposed to intensive training of this kind and learned to maintain wrist stabilization for grasp while she brought the hand to the mouth. Prior to flexing the elbow, and while both hands were in the lap, she used her normal hand to "set" the wrist in extension, because tension in the wrist flexor muscles tended to return.

Hyperactive Wrist Extensor Muscles

In exceptional cases the intensity of automatic wrist extension on fist closure is greatly exaggerated, and wrist extension is so firmly linked with the extensor synergy that, as long as the elbow remains extended, the patient is unable to let the hand drop when he ceases making a fist. In such cases, inhibition of the tense muscles is facilitated if the elbow is passively flexed by the physical therapist. In the flexed position, as the commands "Squeeze" and "Stop squeezing" are given, the patient is instructed not to employ too much force in closing the fist. Practice in relaxation proceeds from the elbow flexed to the elbow extended position.

RELEASE OF GRASP AND EXTENSOR REFLEXES

Although it is true that voluntary grasp needs strengthening, voluntary release of grasp is of equal importance. Spasticity of the flexor muscles of the fingers frequently results in the hand posture seen in Figure 1-10, that is, the thumb is held flexed in the palm of the hand and the other fingers close tightly over the thumb. The spasticity may become so marked that, as the attendant of one male patient said, "I can't pry the hand open." Of course, *prying* the hand open is the wrong approach; there are better ways to release tension in the finger flexor muscles.

A series of manipulations may be performed by the physical therapist to release tension in the flexor muscles of the fingers. These manipulations also tend to transfer some tension to the extensor muscles. When spasticity is present and as long as the patient has no control of finger extension, active grasp must alternate with passive manipulations for release of tension. The patient may learn to carry out some of these manipulations himself and must be made to understand the importance of releasing tension in the spastic flexor muscles. The indiscriminate use of a rubber ball in the affected hand, presumably for strengthening the grip, must be discouraged as it may do more harm than good.

The patient, seen in Figure 3-10, had a right-sided spastic hemiparesis and a great

deal of tension in the flexor muscles of wrist and fingers. A series of manipulations to release tension in her spastic hand muscles is illustrated in Figure 3-11.

First Stage of Manipulations

The patient and the therapist are seated facing each other. The thumb is pulled out of the palm by a grip around the thenar eminence (Fig. 3-11A) and the forearm is supinated (Fig. 3-11B). The therapist's grip is such as to move the thumb at its base joint—movements at the distal thumb joints alone are not very effective. When tension in the flexor muscles is marked, the wrist is allowed to remain in some flexion, as seen in Figure 3-11B. The grasp around the thumb is maintained throughout the manipulations in Figure 3-11A through F; it is perhaps best seen in Figure 3-11D.

The physical therapist now supinates and pronates the patient's forearm repeatedly, emphasizing supination. The pressure on the thumb is lessened when the forearm is pronated and increased during supination. Cutaneous stimulation over the dorsum of wrist and hand is given while the patient's forearm is in the supinated position.

This manipulation, if properly performed and repeated, is usually quite effective in releasing tension in the flexor muscles; simultaneously, some tension appears to develop in the extensor muscles of the fingers. The hand opens up and the fingers extend, partly or fully. If and when a background tension has been evoked in the extensor muscles, the patient may actively participate in opening the hand in the supinated position. However, his effort must be *very slight* because if he tries to force extension he may find that the fingers begin to flex instead. When active finger extension materializes (which is to be differentiated from "tendon action" owing to passive wrist flexion), one may assume that an adequate innervation has resulted from a summation of voluntary and reflex impulses.

Many patients learn to manipulate their own hand in the above manner. This manipulation may be sufficient to bring out complete finger extension, although without it the patient may have little or no control over finger extension. When a patient with right-sided involvement performs manipulations on his own, as in Figure 3-12, he grasps his right thumb with his left hand, pulls the thumb out of the palm and supinates the forearm. Supination of the forearm must be complete so that the patient can look into the palm on the affected side; the normal hand and wrist should make contact with the dorsum of the affected hand. The grip around the thenar eminence of the thumb is maintained during pronation and intensified during supination. Active finger extension, when present, may be reinforced by resistance offered by rubber bands, as illustrated in Figure 3-12*B* and *C*.

Second Stage of Manipulations

If by the above procedure only relative release of tension in the flexor muscles of the fingers has been obtained, additional manipulations are in order. These consist of eliciting stretch reflexes in the finger extensor muscles to further aid in the transfer of tension to these muscles.

As before, the therapist sits facing the patient. When the thumb has been pulled out of the hand and the forearm has been supinated, the therapist uses his free hand for rapid, distally directed stroking movements over the proximal phalanges of the patient's affected hand, thereby causing the metacarpophalangeal joints to flex momentarily (Fig. 3-11*C*) then bounce

FIGURE 3-10. Eleven months after cerebral vascular accident, this patient displayed marked spasticity of wrist and finger flexor muscles on the affected (right) side. The photo was taken prior to the manipulations shown in Figure 3-11. The left side is unaffected, but the hand has a peculiar position. Imitation synkinesis?

back into partial extension. Gradually, the stroking movement is performed in such a manner that first the proximal, then the distal, interphalangeal joints are included. At this time contact with the patient's fingers becomes continuous while a vigorous "rolling" movement is performed causing a rapid flexion and bounce-back at all three finger joints. It is as though the patient's fingertips were drawn to the physical therapist's moving hand by a magnet. The passive finger movements are now extremely rapid and must be performed without interruption. During this manipulation, the patient's finger joints become fully extended, or nearly so, as seen in Figure 3-11*D*, but no tension can be felt in the flexor muscles of the fingers even though these muscles are being rapidly elongated.

The absence of stretch reflexes in the previously spastic finger flexor muscles may be interpreted as resulting from the rapidly repeated stretch reflexes elicited in the *extensor muscles* of the fingers, because when the extensor muscles

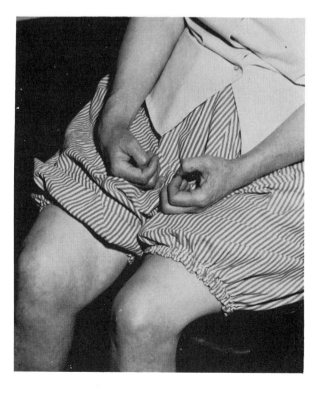

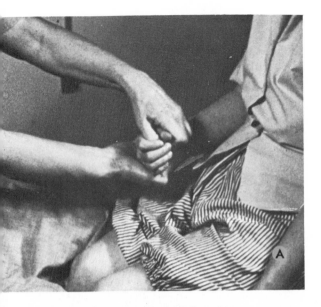

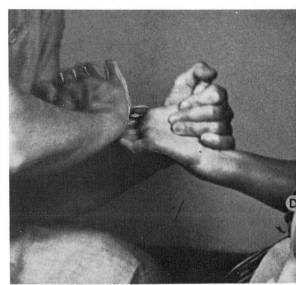

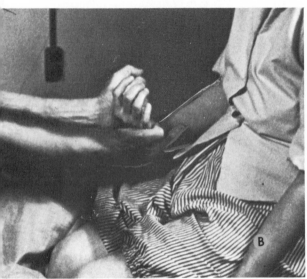

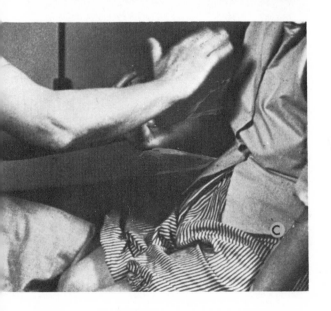

FIGURE 3-11. Techniques used to transfer tension from flexor to extensor muscles. (Frames of a motion picture.) *A.* Thumb is pulled out of the palm of the hand. *B.* Forearm is supinated and dorsum of wrist stimulated. *C.* A stroking movement over the dorsum of the proximal phalanges, which momentarily flexes the metacarpophalangeal joints, is carried out. This frame shows end of stroke. *D.* A rapid "rolling" movement is in progress, causing flexion of all three finger joints (see text). *E.* The physical therapist has risen and made an about-face while maintaining the grip around the patient's thumb and pronating the forearm. Flexor tension is much reduced. *F.* Stroking over the interphalangeal joints begins. *G.* The grip around the thumb has been released. Stroking continues. *H.* The grip around the patient's fingertips has been released. All digits exhibit tonic extension.

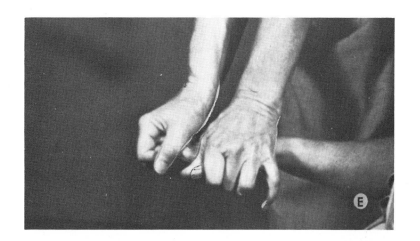

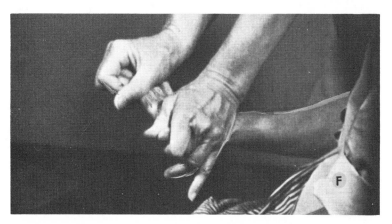

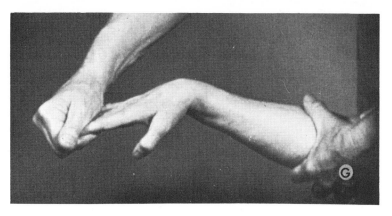

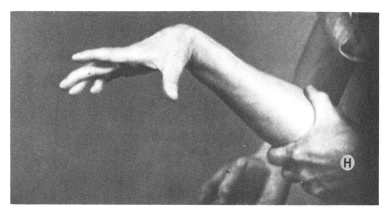

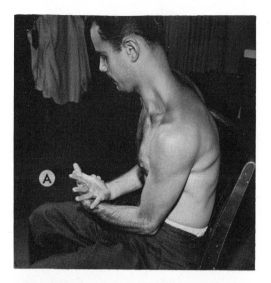

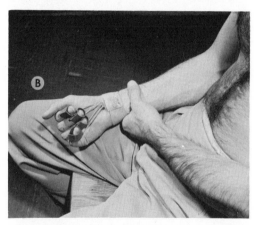

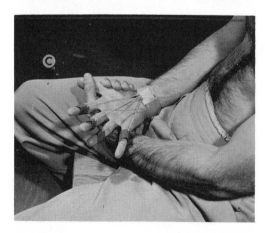

FIGURE 3-12. A 23-year-old patient with right-sided hemiparesis of traumatic origin, 5 years following a head injury. *A.* Voluntary finger extension is facilitated by thumb manipulations and supination of forearm. *B* and *C.* Resistance to finger extension is supplied by rubber bands attached to an outrigger from a wrist band. (From Brunnstrom, S. Motor behavior of adult hemiplegic patients: Hints for training. *Amer. J. Occup. Ther. 15:6,* 1961.)

respond, the flexor muscles are inhibited. However, if stroking is performed over the *palmar* surfaces of the digits, hyperactive stretch reflexes of the flexor muscles return and the fingers bounce back into flexion.

If the position of the patient's wrist in Figure 3-11*D* is compared with that in Figure 3-11*B*, it is obvious that the originally strong tension in the muscles that flex the wrist has also subsided.

Third Stage of Manipulations

The third stage includes elevation of the arm above the horizontal position and the evoking of tonic extensor reflexes of the digits.

After tension in the flexor muscles of the digits has been reduced by the previously described manipulations, the patient's affected forearm is pronated, and the digits are kept fully extended by pressure over the interphalangeal joints and stabilization of the fingertips by the physical therapist; the therapist's left hand maintains its grip around the patient's thumb and also exerts light pressure on the dorsum of the wrist. To accomplish this the therapist must rise and make an about-face so that he comes to stand on the patient's right side (Fig. 3-11*E* and *F*).

The grip around the patient's thumb is now released and the arm is raised above the horizontal position. The therapist performs distally directed stroking movements over the interphalangeal joints with the heel of the hand (Fig. 3-11*F* and *G*). Any tension that may remain in or may have returned to the finger flexor muscles disappears as a result of stimulation over the dorsum of the fingers. It appears as if the joints were "molded" into an extended, even hyperextended, position (Fig. 3-11*G*). The joints will maintain this position as the therapist gently slides his hand in a distal direction and discontinues the contact with the patient's hand (Fig. 3-11*H*).

The reflex that has just been evoked has a tonic character. Reinforcement of the reflex is obtained if the fingers are passively flexed by stroking over the extensor side of the hand and digits. Following such passive flexion the fingers bounce back to the extended positions. During the entire procedure the patient remains inactive but observes what happens to the hand. When the patient is ready, voluntary impulses are superimposed on the reflex; additional extension of the digits may then be observed. As before, the patient's voluntary effort must be slight, not much more than a mental effort.

Figure 3-13 shows the effect of manipulations and arm elevation on another patient whose fist was habitually so strongly closed that, according to his attendant, he was unable to wash the inside of the hand. The attendant learned to manipulate the patient's hand and reported good results.

The Tonic Thumb Reflex

The tonic thumb reflex is closely related to the general extension reflex discussed above in the preceding section. The response of the thumb becomes intensified if the forearm is supinated when the arm is elevated. The hand should reach at least the height of the forehead, preferably positioned overhead, as in Figure 3-14. The reflex develops slowly; several seconds are required before it reaches its maximum. Index extension often accompanies the thumb response, but the behavior of this finger varies in individuals. The intensity of the reflex response is augmented if each finger is passively flexed, then is allowed to rebound (Fig. 3-14).

In some patients an elevation of the arm together with supination of the forearm suffices to evoke the reflex, but for most patients it is advisable first to manipulate the hand to decrease tension in the flexor muscles.

Few patients demonstrate a fully developed reflex as seen in Figure 3-14, but in most cases the arm position illustrated appears to *facilitate* a voluntary thumb movement and is therefore useful for training purposes.

To facilitate *extension of the fourth and fifth fingers* the forearm should remain

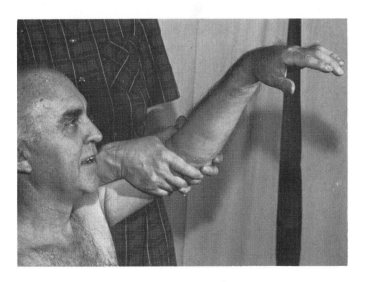

FIGURE 3-13. A 54-year-old man with left-sided hemiparesis of 14 months' duration. The hand was mostly firmly closed, thumb in palm, as seen in Figure 1-10. Tonic finger extension resulted from hand manipulations and elevation of the arm. (From Brunnstrom, S. Motor behavior of adult hemiplegic patients: Hints for training. *Amer. J. Occup. Ther.* 15:6, 1961.)

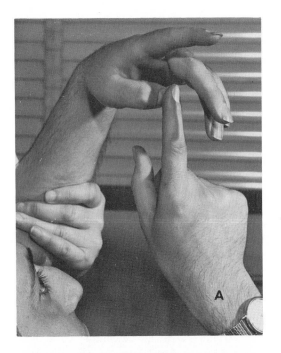

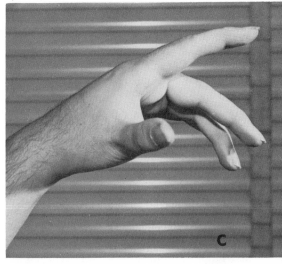

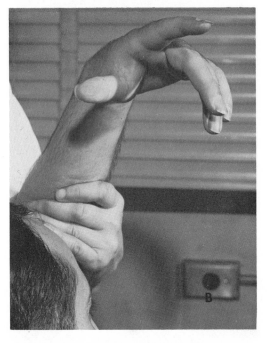

FIGURE 3-14. Tonic thumb and index extension reflex in 30-year-old man with left-sided hemiparesis resulting from a head injury. *A* and *B*. Amplitude of thumb reflex is increased if the thumb is passively flexed, then allowed to rebounce. *C*. Rebound of index finger following passive flexion of this finger. (From Brunnstrom, S. Motor behavior of adult hemiplegic patients: Hints for training. *Amer. J. Occup. Ther. 15:6*, 1961.)

whether friction is carried out in a distal direction only or by rubbing up and down the forearm.

ALTERNATE FIST CLOSURE AND FIST OPENING

When the extensor reflexes of the digits have been well established, the arm is passively lowered and the elbow flexed; the forearm and the wrist are supported. In this position, the patient is requested to make a fist, but the command "Squeeze" is followed by "Stop squeezing" as soon as the fingers begin to flex. Without delay the arm is then raised to its previous position. Under favorable conditions, the tonic extensor response then reappears. The patient observes how the fingers extend and "thinks" extension. He has been informed that he may voluntarily assist extension if he feels that he is ready for it but that extension must not be forced. The

pronated as the arm is elevated. Intensive friction over the ulnar side of the dorsum of the forearm further reinforces the voluntary effort, which was the case of the patient in Figure 3-15. When providing friction, the physical therapist may use the dorsal or palmar side of his fingertips, or his knuckles, and it appears immaterial

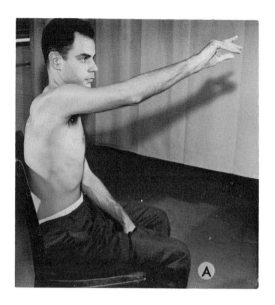

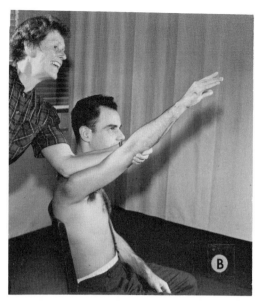

FIGURE 3-15. A 23-year-old patient with right-sided spastic hemiparesis. *A.* Maximal voluntary finger extension with arm elevated. *B.* Following friction over the ulnar aspect of the dorsum of the forearm (and support of the arm), increased range of finger extension is obtained.

alternation between finger flexion and finger extension, if properly timed, appears to reinforce extension. Possibly, the mechanism of successive induction is responsible for such reinforcement (see Sherrington, 1947 p. 209).

At this stage, when finger extension is essentially a reflex phenomenon or occurs as the result of an interaction between voluntary and reflex impulses, the patient is not expected to grasp and release objects placed in the hand, which requires further progress.

After the voluntary component of fist opening with the arm held elevated has been strengthened, the patient must learn to open the fist in gradually lowered positions. As before, fist opening alternates with fist closure. If excessive tension in the finger flexor muscles returns, manipulations are repeated.

The ability of a patient to open the hand in the elevated position of the arm

before being able to do so in other arm positions is no doubt related to Souques' phenomenon, discussed in Chapter 1.

SENSATIONS WHICH PRECEDE OR ACCOMPANY VOLUNTARY FINGER EXTENSION

Judging from unsolicited remarks by patients with hemiparesis specific sensations appear to be precursors of voluntary control of movement. Such sensations are probably most marked in relation to movements of the hand and specifically of the fingers.

One patient (Fig. 3-14) who had strong voluntary fist closure but who was unable to extend the fingers experienced very different sensations with respect to finger extension, depending on the posture of the arm. When the arm was passively held in the elevated position, he said, "I know that I will be able to extend the fingers myself any moment now." But when the hand was in his lap, he commented, "In this position, I cannot even *think* of opening the fist."

Another patient demonstrated his ability to extend the fingers for part of the range when he held the forearm supinated and the elbow flexed to an obtuse angle when the hand was just off his lap. As an experiment, the physical therapist pronated the forearm and asked the patient to extend the fingers. "Impossible," the patient replied. "In that position the fingers are locked."

In the case of a young woman with hemiparesis, it was discovered that she had good control of mass finger extension when the physical therapist held the arm in a forward-downward direction, elbow extended and forearm pronated. Other arm postures were experimented with but brought little or no success. The posture which in this patient best facilitated finger extension was used a number of times during each training session. It must have given the patient a special sensation because one day she spontaneously exclaimed, "My hand just *adores* this position!"

Favorable sensations are often experienced by patients following certain manipulations and after cutaneous stimuli have been applied. What the patient feels he cannot always find words for, but his facial expression unmistakably indicates that something has happened; perhaps he experiences a sensation that has long been lost, which tells him that changes to the better have taken place. He appears to anticipate a movement that he has not yet been able to master.

TRANSITION TO VOLUNTARY FINGER EXTENSION

During training sessions, the physical therapist must prepare the patient for voluntary finger extension by releasing tension in the finger flexor muscles and by evoking a background tension in the extensor muscles. Manipulations, surface stimulation, favorable body position, and arm positioning are examples of procedures that may produce the desired results. When favorable conditions for finger extension have been set up, voluntary extension may materialize. But as long as a voluntary

impulse needs specific reflex reinforcement to acquire threshold intensity, the ensuing movement must be classified as *semivoluntary*.

Semivoluntary Mass Extension of Digits

Results obtained from preparatory procedures and favorable arm positioning are seen in Figure 3-16, which are frames of a motion picture taken during a training session. Although every patient cannot be expected to respond in the same manner and with the same vigor, this patient demonstrated some general principles that should be kept in mind.

Seven weeks following a cerebral vascular accident, the patient was able to make a firm fist with the arm in any position, but she could not extend the fingers by voluntary effort alone. The influence of the basic limb synergies had been strong during several weeks after the stroke, then such influence began to decline, as evident from her ability to raise the arm to a forward-horizontal position without difficulty. After having closed the hand, however, she could release the grasp only slightly, using a small range extension movement at the metacarpophalangeal joints; the interphalangeal joints remained flexed (Fig. 3-16A). Her effort to extend the fingers is reflected in her facial expression and by "imitation synkinesis" of the hand on the normal side.

The patient's ability to extend the fingers improved if the therapist supported the arm and lowered it a little from the position seen in Figure 3-16A; the additional extension movement occurred mainly at the metacarpophalangeal joints. A remarkable improvement in finger extension was obtained in the arm positions seen in Figure 3-16B and C. Note that in the side-horizontal position, the patient's forearm is fully pronated and that extension is most marked in the fourth and fifth fingers. As the therapist switched to the overhead position and supinated the forearm, the extension response was again good, but this time the thumb and the index finger responded best. In both positions, not only the fist but also the mouth opened up in a synkinetic imitation movement.

Judging from this patient's responses and from similar responses of other patients in approximately the same recovery stages, semivoluntary finger extension is notably influenced by the posture of the limb as a whole; that is, it is linked to certain gross movements of the limb other than the basic limb synergies. The two limb postures illustrated are in fact end positions of two opposite movement combinations. The overhead position combines a forward movement of the scapula, external rotation of the shoulder, supination of the forearm, and extension of the digits, most marked in the fingers on the radial side. In the side-horizontal position, the movement direction at all joints has been reversed, as compared to the overhead position; the scapula is retracted, the shoulder internally rotated, the forearm pronated, the wrist ulnar-flexed; finger extension is most marked in the fingers on the ulnar side.

Individual Thumb Movements

In the case of the patient seen in Figure 3-16, voluntary thumb movements began to appear at the time when semivoluntary mass extension became possible. Following manipulations to release tension in the flexor muscles of the fingers and with the

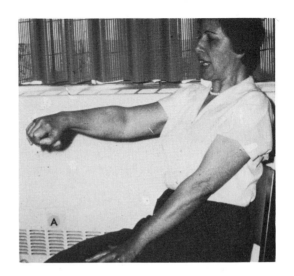

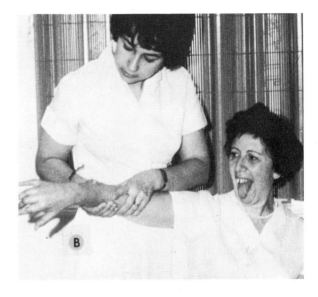

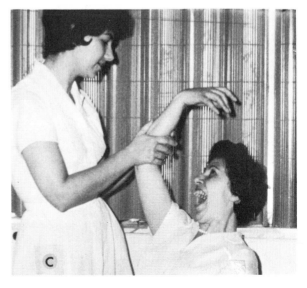

FIGURE 3-16. A 52-year-old woman with right-sided hemiparesis, 7 weeks after a stroke. (Frames of a motion picture.) *A.* With the arm in the forward-horizontal position, the patient is able to open the fist only slightly. Note facial expression and fist opening on normal side. *B.* With the arm supported in the side-horizontal position, forearm fully pronated, finger extension is facilitated, markedly so in the fourth and fifth fingers. *C.* The overhead position favors thumb and index extension.

hand placed in the lap, ulnar side down, the patient was capable of moving the thumb away from contact with the index finger (Fig. 3-17). Control of this movement is considered particularly important because it is a requirement for learning lateral prehension, a type of grasp that the stroke patient can use for numerous functional activities.

When the patient first attempts to move the thumb away from the other fingers he must make only a minimal effort, because if he tries to force the movement the thumb as well as the other fingers will begin to flex. If the patient needs assistance, the therapist may stimulate the tendons of the abductor pollicis longus and the extensor pollicis brevis muscles where they pass over the wrist by gentle local percussion or by friction in the same area.

For lateral prehension it does not make much difference in what direction the thumb moves, as long as it moves away from the other digits. For further control of thumb movements, the patient learns to "twiddle" his thumbs. He folds his hands allowing some flexion of the wrists and moves the two thumbs around each other.

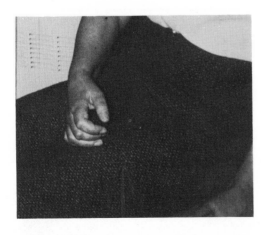

FIGURE 3-17. Same person as in Figure 3-16, 7 weeks following the stroke. The thumb can be separated from the index finger for only a short distance. The available thumb movement suffices for grasp and release of small objects using lateral prehension. (Frame of a motion picture.)

At first, the thumb on the normal side may have to push the other one around, but if the patient concentrates the other thumb may soon begin to participate. It may be assumed that the willed effort, together with visual guidance and sensory impulses from both the affected and the unaffected sides, may combine to bring out the coordination required for this movement.

As long as extension movements of the digits are semivoluntary, the patient must be comfortably relaxed and feel at ease during all training sessions. Excessive tension in muscles throughout the affected limb and the body as a whole must be avoided or finger extension will not materialize. This is one of the reasons why the physical therapist should carry the involved limb and move it from one position to the other. In Figure 3-16A the patient held the arm up herself, which required muscular effort, and she was not very successful in releasing the grasp. But when the therapist supported the arm in almost the same position, release of grasp improved. The semivoluntary finger extension, seen in Figure 3-16B and C, would not have succeeded if the weight of the arm had not been carried by the physical therapist.

VOLUNTARY FINGER EXTENSION

Unfortunately, many patients with hemiplegia never reach the advanced recovery stages during which voluntary finger extension becomes possible. However, once semivoluntary finger extension has been established, chances are good that voluntary extension will follow so that the patient can open and close the hand in all arm postures and without preliminary preparation. This was true of the patient seen in Figures 2-5B and C and 2-6.

PREHENSION TYPES

In Chapter 2, on page 2 of the evaluation form, common prehension types are listed in the order of their difficulties for patients with hemiplegia.

Hook Grasp

Hook grasp requires that the patient has control of fist closure, not necessarily fist opening, and that the grasp is sufficiently strong to hold on to the handles of a hand-bag or light briefcase. The patient may have to use the normal hand to place the handles in the affected hand, then make a conscious effort to maintain a firm grip. The affected hand may thus be of use when the patient wishes to free his normal hand for a more complicated job, such as turning a door knob and opening a door. However, it may not be practical for the patient to use the hook grasp to hold an object when walking, because when his attention is focused elsewhere the handles may slip out of the hand without the patient noticing it. The inability of a patient with hemiplegia to maintain a grip without conscious effort, as one would normally do, is probably because of deficient sensation, which is so often present in these patients.

Lateral Prehension

For this type of grasp, the patient must be able to maintain the thumb outside of the palm of the hand and to move it a short distance away from the index finger when approaching an object. The grasp is accomplished by pressure of the thumb against the radial side of the index finger. Because no portion of the object comes in contact with the palm of the hand, release is comparatively easy.

Normally, lateral prehension is performed with the interphalangeal joint of the thumb extended and used mainly for grasping small, rather flat objects. When the patient with hemiplegia first acquires the ability to use lateral prehension, he may still possess only mass grasp, therefore the interphalangeal joint of the thumb

tends to flex. This, however, does not detract from its usefulness for grasping small objects, for adjusting clothing, and for a variety of other tasks.

A prime requirement for lateral prehension is a degree of individual thumb control, which explains why so much emphasis is placed on the thumb reflex at an early date—it is hoped that semivoluntary and voluntary movements will follow. The patient in Figure 3-17, seven weeks following a cerebral vascular accident, had learned to move the thumb away from the other fingers and soon began to use lateral prehension, although awkwardly, for functional activities. Many more weeks were required before she acquired the ability to use more advanced prehension types.

Advanced Prehension

In general, the requirements for advanced prehension types are as follows: (1) Voluntary fist opening; (2) opposition of the thumb toward the other fingers; and (3) the ability to release objects in contact with the palmar side of the hand.

After discharge from the Neurological Institute the patient in Figure 3-17 continued training in an out-patient clinic and made gradual progress in the use of her hand. She was not seen by the author until about six months following her cerebral vascular accident, when new motion pictures were taken.

At this time, synergy influence had completely disappeared and no spasticity could be detected. She opened her hand without preliminary preparation; that is, she had advanced from semivoluntary to voluntary finger extension (Fig. 3-18*A*). She opposed her thumb to any one of the other digits but experienced some difficulty in reaching the tip of her little finger (Fig. 3-18*B* and *C*); contact with the palm of the hand no longer prevented release of objects. *Palmar prehension* was used to grasp and release a pencil (Fig. 2-10), *cylindrical grasp* for holding and releasing a mug (Fig. 2-11),

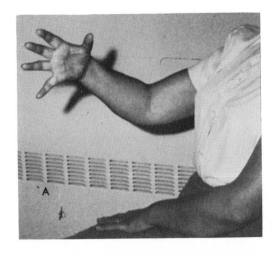

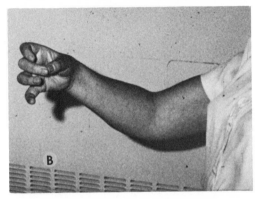

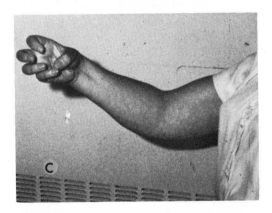

FIGURE 3-18. Same person as in Figures 3-16 and 3-17, 6 months after the stroke. (Frames of a motion picture.) *A.* Voluntary fist opening, full range. Exaggerated finger abduction may have resulted from the patient's effort to extend the fingers maximally. *B* and *C.* Opposition of thumb to third and fifth fingers.

and *spherical grasp* for holding and releasing a ball (Fig. 2-12). She was also able to throw the ball with fair accuracy, which necessitates rapid release and coordinated motion throughout the upper limb.

FUNCTIONAL HAND ACCOMPLISHMENTS

Lateral Prehension Present. A patient must not necessarily master advanced prehension types before being able to function well with respect to most ordinary two-handed activities. For example, the patient seen in Figure 3-19 learned to perform a variety of activities with the use of thumb pressure against the other digits, although she had little if any control of the opposition movement. When grasping and holding an object, the interphalangeal joint of the thumb invariably flexed because the mechanism of mass grasp prevailed. The patient was able to disengage the grip of the thumb sufficiently to release small objects, but for larger objects she had to use her normal hand to disengage the object. Two-handed activities, which were documented by motion pictures (in addition to the ones seen in Figure 3-19) included the following: stabilizing a piece of meat with an ordinary fork while the normal hand was used to cut the meat; holding a saltshaker while unscrewing its top with the normal hand; holding a matchbook while striking a match with the normal hand; stabilizing a glass while pouring water from a pitcher; and carrying a tray full of dishes to the kitchen. She also used her affected hand for bringing a piece of bread to the mouth and, without difficulty, wiped her mouth with a paper napkin, also with the affected hand.

Advanced Prehension Present. The patient seen in Figure 3-18 gained control of advanced prehension types. She acquired a degree of finger dexterity, which she used for tying her shoelaces (with both hands),

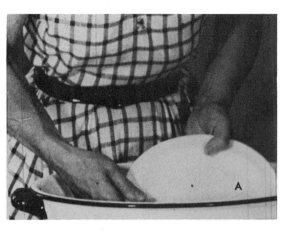

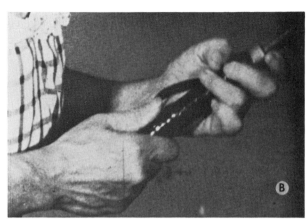

FIGURE 3-19. Patient with left-sided hemiparesis using the available thumb movement in washing dishes (*A*) and in opening an umbrella (*B*) (see text). (Frames of a motion picture.)

for various household activities, and for knitting with large needles. She also proudly demonstrated that, using her affected hand only, she could button and unbutton her blouse which had small buttons (Fig. 3-20). Understandably, she preferred to use her normal hand for this activity because the affected hand was less skillful and rather slow in accomplishing the task. Individual thumb movements were present

in all directions, and when she grasped an object in the hand she experienced no difficulty keeping the interphalangeal joint of the thumb extended—she had advanced well beyond the stage of mass grasp. Voluntary complete finger extension enabled her to release objects of any size. Isolated movements of the second to fifth fingers were also present, but they were not as well performed as on the normal side.

There was no opportunity to examine this patient at a later date, and therefore it is not known whether the hand continued to improve. Nor is it known whether 6 months of uninterrupted training was at least in part responsible for her spectacular improvement. Possibly, such improvement would have occurred spontaneously without organized training.

The carefully documented story of this patient, however, clearly shows that she went through all sequential recovery stages outlined in Chapter 2, and that in her case 6 months were required to reach Stage 6, at which time control of all proximal joints was normal and hand control was well advanced, even though the hand still lacked skill.

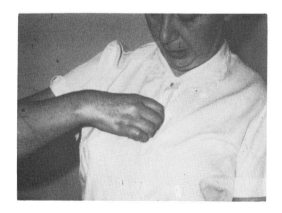

FIGURE 3-20. Same person as in Figure 3-18, 6 months following a stroke. She managed, with some difficulty, to button and unbutton her blouse, using the affected hand only. (Frame of a motion picture.)

REFERENCES

BASMAJIAN, J. V. *Muscles Alive*, 2nd ed. Baltimore, William & Wilkins, 1966, pp. 168–172.

BRAIN, W. R. The significance of the flexor posture of the upper limb in hemiplegia, with an account of a quadrupedal extensor reflex. *Brain* 50:113, 1927.

EGEL, P. *Technique of Treatment for the Cerebral Palsy Child.* St. Louis, Mosby, 1948, p. 118.

FAY, T. The use of pathological and unlocking reflexes in the rehabilitation of spastics. *Amer. J. Phys. Med.* 33:347, 1954.

JACKSON, J. H. "Evolution and Dissolution of the Nervous System" (1884), in *Selected Writings of John Hughlings Jackson,* ed. by J. Taylor. New York, Basic Books, 1958, pp. 45–75.

MAGNUS, R. Some results of studies in the physiology of posture, Part 1, *Lancet 211 (2):*531, 1926.

MAGNUS, R., and DE KLEIJN, A. Die Abhängigkeit des Tonus der Extremitätenmuskeln von der Kopfstellung. *Pflüger Arch. Physiol.* 45:455, 1912.

MARIE, P., and FOIX, C. Les syncinécies des hémiplégiques. *Rev. Neurol.* 29:3, and 30:145, 1916.

PHELPS, W. The care and treatment of cerebral palsies. *J. Amer. Med. Ass.* 111:1, 1938.

SHERRINGTON, C. S. *The Integrative Action of the Nervous System,* 2nd ed., New Haven, Yale Univ. Press, 1947, p. 209.

As an introduction to training procedures for the lower limb, a discussion of gait patterns in patients with hemiplegia is presented here. Because weight bearing and walking are the most important functions of the lower limbs, training must be oriented toward restoring safe standing and the ability to walk safely in as normal a manner as possible.

A study of the hemiplegic gait begins with a comparison between the phasic action of muscles in normal locomotion and the muscle combinations characteristic of the primitive movement synergies of flexion and extension. After this comparison has been made, there is the challenging task of finding ways and means of modifying the gross movement synergies to bring about muscle combinations resembling, if not identical with, those employed in normal walking.

Walking patterns of normal individuals are now reasonably well known with respect both to joint movement and muscular activity. Under standardized conditions, these patterns vary only a little among individuals (Eberhart, Inman, and associates, 1947). Gait patterns of patients with hemiplegia, on the other hand, are quite variable depending upon the severity of the involvement and the manner of compensation that the patient employs.

The gait patterns of eleven patients who had sustained cerebral vascular accidents were investigated by Hirschberg and Nathanson (1952). The study revealed that considerable changes in the phasic action of muscles, as compared to muscle action in normal walking, had occurred. The changes also involved the normal limb. This was to be expected since the normal limb must make major adjustments when the affected limb fails to perform properly. That the patients selected for this study had relatively mild involvement may be concluded from the records that show heel-toe gait and marked activity of the tibialis anterior muscle in swing phase.

Gait Patterns in Hemiplegia

The study confirmed a number of common clinical observations: that the stance phase on the affected side of these patients is considerably shorter, and the swing phase correspondingly longer, than on the normal side; that the quadriceps and the gastrocnemius muscles on the paretic side are active throughout stance phase; and that all muscle groups on the nonparetic side intensify their activity, as compared to normal gait.

The electromyograms from this study also indicated that the gluteus maximus and the semitendinosus muscles on the affected side contracted throughout stance phase, characteristics that would be difficult to observe clinically. It is also interesting that the phasic action of muscles of the nonparetic limb showed considerable resemblance with that of the paretic limb.

To the author's knowledge, extensive objective records of kinematic and kinetic aspects of hemiplegic locomotion of patients with varying degree of involvement and utilizing different types of compensation are not available. However, the energy cost of hemiparetic, as compared to nonparetic, patients during walking at different speeds was studied by Bard (1963), and the effect on energy expenditure during walking while wearing a brace was studied by Bard and Ralston (1959).

CLINICAL RECORDING OF GAIT FOR PATIENTS WITH HEMIPLEGIA

The method of recording gait used by the author is essentially a subjective one, inasmuch as it does not use instrumentation. Its lack of true objectivity is by far outweighed by its practical aspects; no time-consuming preparations are needed, very little space is required, and it is easy to administer. The experienced observer can evaluate and record the gait without the patient's knowing that he is being "tested," which has definite advantages. By systematically observing the behavior of the three main weight-bearing joints—an-

kle, knee, and hip—specific data are collected which, when put together, furnish a rather complete picture of the patient's gait.

The detailed gait analysis form presented here (Chart 2), which is designed for the evaluation of level walking only, lists various commonly found gait deviations. The faulty gait components are listed to draw the examiner's attention to deficiencies at the three main weight-bearing joints. The same gait analysis procedure is intended to be used on the main evaluation form (Chapter 2), but on this form the faulty components have to be written in, which requires that the examiner be familiar with the common walking difficulties of patients with hemiplegia.

Some of the components listed on the form can only be properly recorded if the patient is capable of walking without a cane and without a brace. If the patient uses walking aids, this must be indicated. A gait analysis of very severely affected patients is not attempted.

Figures 4-1 and 4-2, which illustrate certain aspects of the kinematics and kinetics of normal gait, should be consulted freely during the discussion that follows, particularly by those readers who are not familiar with the locomotion study by Eberhart, Inman, and Associates (1947). The vertical lines in Figure 4-1 indicate heel contact, ball contact, ball rise, and toe off, respectively, of one limb. In Figure 4-2 only those vertical lines that represent heel contact and toe off are shown. The contralateral limb is not included in these two illustrations, i.e., the period of double stance when both feet are on the ground is not indicated.

MUSCLE ACTION IN NORMAL WALKING COMPARED WITH THAT OF THE LIMB SYNERGIES

The curves in Figure 4-2 show that at no time during the walking cycle do the muscles act in combinations identical with

Chart 2

HEMIPLEGIA—GAIT ANALYSIS

Name_____   Evaluation date_____

Ankle: Stance Phase

Entire sole down_____

Toes first_____

Inversion, early stance_____

Inversion throughout_____

Affected foot leads_____

Heel-toe action near normal_____

_____

Knee: Stance Phase

Knee buckles_____

Hyperextension, mild_____

Hyperextension, moderate_____

Hyperextension, severe_____

Stable in slight flexion_____

Near normal_____

_____

Hip: Stance Phase

Trendelenburg_____

Trunk forward_____

Stable, near normal_____

_____

_____

Ankle: Swing Phase

Toes dragging_____

Inversion_____

Exaggerated dorsiflexion_____

"Whip"_____

Eversion_____

_____

Knee: Swing Phase

Stiff_____

Moderately stiff_____

Free, near normal_____

Exaggerated flexion_____

_____

Hip: Swing Phase

Circumduction_____

Pelvic hike_____

Stiff (pelvic tilt)_____

Moderately stiff_____

Free, near normal_____

Exaggerated flexion_____

External rotation_____

_____

those of the basic limb synergies. When these limb synergies dominate the motor behavior, the activation of muscle groups in combinations and sequences required for normal walking is prevented.

The electromyograms of normal walking also indicate that a rapid rise and fall in tension of the muscle groups is required. In contrast, when the basic limb synergies are activated, muscular tension is slow in building up and slow in fading out.

In general, it may be stated that the difficulties encountered by patients with hemiplegia are related to two main factors: firm linkage of muscle groups in accordance with the dictum of primitive movement synergies, and slowness of reactions of muscle groups.

The gait analysis form provides space for recording the behavior of ankle, knee, and hip on the affected side during stance phase and swing phase. The items listed

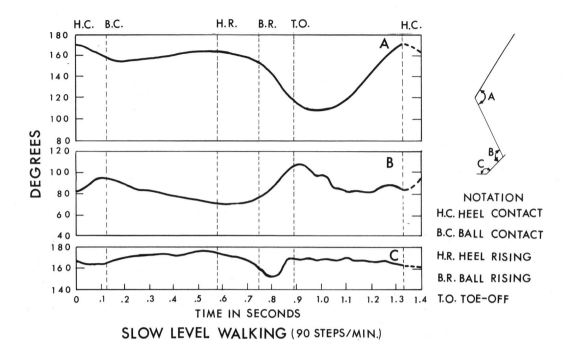

FIGURE 4-1. Angles between leg and foot segments during level walking at 90 steps per minute. (Redrawn from Fig. 4-23 in Eberhart, H. D., Inman, V. T., and Associates. *Report to the National Research Council, Committee on Artificial Limbs, on Fundamental Studies of Human Locomotion and Other Information Relating to Design of Artificial Limbs.* University of California, Berkeley, 1947, Vol. I.)

all have been observed clinically, although with varying frequency.

ANKLE JOINT: STANCE PHASE

For the present discussion it is convenient to speak about early stance, midstance, and late stance because the forces acting on the supporting limb change significantly in the course of the weight-bearing phase. No attempts have been made to define these subdivisions in terms of percentage of the walking cycle.

Early Stance, Normal Gait. As the heel strikes the ground at the beginning of stance phase, the angle between the foot and the leg (angle B, Fig. 4-1) is approximately 90 degrees. As weight is shifted to the forward foot, the sole of the foot is gradually and smoothly lowered to the ground. During this phase, only minor changes in the foot-leg angle occur, owing to the stabilizing action of the muscles which prevent a sudden plantar flexion of the ankle. For this stabilization, the dorsiflexor muscles of the ankle (pretibial group, Fig. 4-2) are responsible; they resist a stretching force caused by the impact of the body weight on the heel.

Early Stance, Hemiplegic Gait. When the basic limb synergies are dominant, anticipation of weight bearing on the affected limb frequently activates all the components of the extensor synergy, including the plantar flexors of the ankle. The tension which is thus set up in the calf muscles maintains the ankle in plantar flexion, and as a result the heel and the ball of the foot make contact with the ground simultaneously. The dorsiflexor muscles of the ankle, being component parts of the flexor synergy, refuse to associate themselves with the knee extensor muscles. On the gait analysis form this condition is described as *entire sole down.* If spasticity is marked, the patient may even touch the ground with the *toes first.* When *inversion* of the ankle is pronounced, the weight will be borne on the outside of the foot, and in that case walking without an ankle brace or other control is not advisable. Many patients, however, display only a moderate amount of *inversion in early stance,* an inversion that corrects itself as the weight is shifted over the foot. In severely involved patients the extensor synergy may set in strongly before the affected foot touches the ground. The adductor component may be so marked that the affected limb draws close to the normal one, or goes into extreme adduction, crossing in front of the normal limb. In that case, weight bearing on the affected limb becomes almost impossible.

Midstance, Normal Gait. When the ball of the foot has made contact with the ground, the task of the dorsiflexor muscles of the ankle has been completed. With the sole firmly on the ground, the leg starts pivoting forward about the ankle joint, causing the foot-leg angle (angle B, Fig. 4-1) to decrease somewhat. As the body weight advances in front of the ankle joint, action of the plantar flexor muscles begins (Fig. 4-2). Excessive forward pivoting of the leg at the ankle is prevented by a lengthening contraction of the calf muscles as these muscles resist the stretching force of the body weight. During this phase, a gradual, controlled, small-range elongation of the calf muscles takes place.

Midstance, Hemiplegic Gait. Spastic muscles are hypersensitive to stretch. When stretched, they respond by increasing their tension. The calf muscles are no exception to this rule. When acted upon by the body weight their tension is reinforced, often to such an extent that no elongation can take place. This prevents forward pivoting of the leg at the ankle and interferes with proper forward motion of the body. The patient finds it difficult to advance the normal foot the proper distance in front of

the affected foot and the strides become unequal. The swing phase of the normal limb is executed too rapidly, which further contributes to the disturbance of the natural walking rhythm. When tension in the calf muscles is marked and unyielding, *the affected foot may lead* all along, so that the patient advances the affected foot, then draws the normal foot up to, but not beyond, the affected one.

Late Stance, Normal Gait. Toward the end of the stance phase, as the limb prepares for the forward swing, the heel rises from the ground and simultaneously the knee begins to flex (Fig. 4-1). At this moment a rapid increase in the tension and peak activity of the calf muscles occurs (Fig. 4-2). In this phase the ankle plantar flexes, and the calf muscles have reversed their action from a lengthening to a shortening contraction. Because the knee extensors at this time are inactive and because the main portion of the body weight is now on the contralateral limb, the push-off of the calf muscles causes the foot to detach itself from the ground as hip and knee flex. Together with other muscular and gravitational forces, the calf muscles thus are instrumental in initiating the forward swing of the limb.

Late Stance, Hemiplegic Gait. The failure of the affected limb to perform properly is particularly noticeable in late stance phase. First, tension in the quadriceps muscles often persists into this phase and prevents the knee from flexing, or causes it to flex too slowly. Second, flexion of the hip and knee together with active push-off by the calf muscles, as required in normal walking, does not materialize; neither the flexor synergy nor the extensor synergy provides this combination. Detachment of the foot becomes difficult, and the forces needed for the initiation of the swing phase are inadequate. The limb therefore has to be brought forward by some compensatory method.

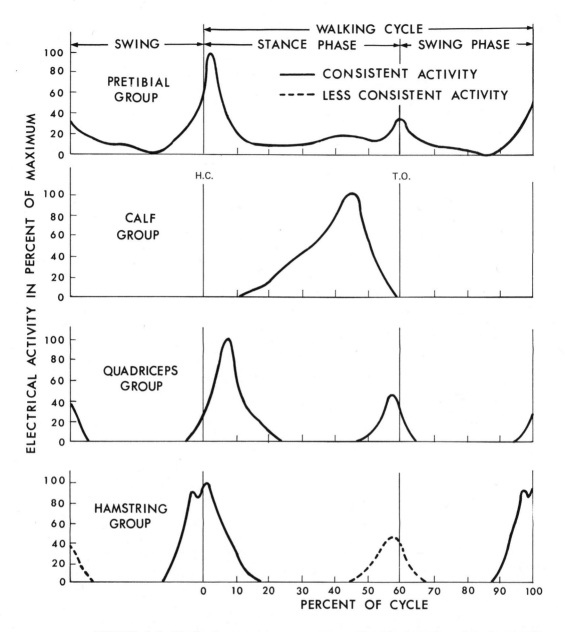

FIGURE 4-2. Idealized summary curves representing phasic action of major muscle groups during level walking, derived from electromyograph studies on 10 adult males walking at 95 steps per minute. (Redrawn from Fig. 3-39 in Eberhart, H. D., Inman, V. T., and Associates. *Report to the National Research Council, Committee on Artificial Limbs, on Fundamental Studies of Human Locomotion and Other Information Relating to Design of Artificial Limbs.* University of California, Berkeley, 1947, Vol. I.)

KNEE JOINT: STANCE PHASE

Early Stance and Midstance, Normal Gait. At the moment when the heel makes contact with the ground, the knee is extended or nearly extended. After heel contact, under the impact of the body weight, a knee flexion of short duration and small range sets in, followed by knee extension (angle A, Fig. 4-1). This flexion-

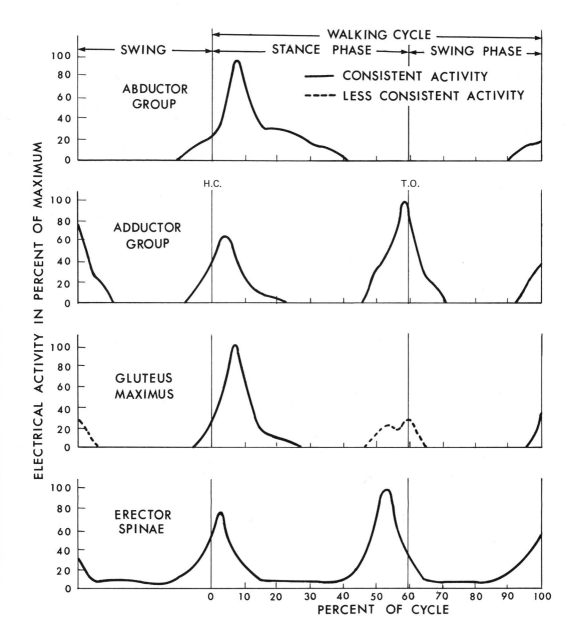

extension movement is instrumental in keeping the path of the center of gravity of the body from rising and falling abruptly, thus aiding a smooth forward translatory movement of the body. The electromyograms show peak activity of the quadriceps muscles during the flexion portion of the knee curve in early stance (Fig. 4-2). Muscular activity thus prevents a buckling of the knee at a time when the body weight acts posteriorly to the knee axis. A sharp drop and complete cessation of activity of the quadriceps muscles follow, indicating that in midstance knee extensor activity is no longer needed.

Early Stance and Midstance, Hemiplegic Gait. If the limb is essentially flaccid, as in the early stage following a stroke, the knee may be incapable of supporting the body weight—that is, the *knee buckles* and a fall may result. (An improvised splint may then be applied until it can be determined if a permanent brace is required to stabilize the knee. Generally, the knee extensor muscles soon become activated upon weight bearing, hence a long leg brace is seldom required.)

A common appearance in this phase of walking is *hyperextension* of the knee at a time when a flexion-extension movement should take place. The hyperextension may be mild, moderate, or severe. Except in totally flaccid cases, weight bearing tends to elicit a contraction in the quadriceps muscles, but these muscles fail to regulate their activity to the requirements of normal gait. A hyperextended knee offers increased stability and is therefore a purposeful compensation for a patient who does not have full knee control. Excessive tension in the calf muscles prevents a forward pivoting of the leg at the ankle, and hyperextension of the knee may occur because the ankle fails to yield.

Some patients show an increased flexion of the knee in early stance and the knee momentarily appears to give, but the knee becomes *stable in slight flexion* and forward weight shift is facilitated. It would seem as if the quadriceps muscles were called into action upon heel contact but perhaps with insufficient speed or strength. As the body weight starts to flex the knee, the quadriceps muscles become stretched, and this stretch reinforces its contraction so that weight bearing on a slightly flexed knee becomes possible.

Late Stance, Normal Gait. In this phase, the knee flexes and the ankle plantar flexes (angles A and B, Fig. 4-1). This requires an inhibition of the quadriceps muscles and a strong activation of the calf muscles (peak contraction, Fig. 4-2). This combination, together with flexion of the hip, initiates the forward swing of the limb.

Late Stance, Hemiplegic Gait. The strong linkage that exists between the calf muscles and the quadriceps muscles in patients with hemiplegia does not allow the muscle combination that is required in late stance phase for normal progression. Preparation for swing phase, as described above, therefore fails, and the patient seeks other ways of moving the affected limb forward.

HIP JOINT: STANCE PHASE

Early Stance and Midstance, Normal Gait. One important requirement at the hip during normal weight bearing is the activation of the abductor muscles of the hip. These muscles provide lateral stabilization of the pelvis, preventing the opposite side of the pelvis from sagging. The hip abductor muscles show peak activity just after heel contact, and they continue being active (with lesser intensity) throughout midstance. The extensor muscles of the hip show a burst of activity after heel contact, an activity that rapidly decreases and ceases before midstance (Fig. 4-2).

Early Stance and Midstance, Hemiplegic Gait. When the extensor synergy is activated upon weight bearing (often in anticipation of weight bearing), the adductor muscles of the hip, together with other components of the extensor synergy, contract. On the other hand, the abductor muscles which belong to the flexor synergy fail to respond, and lateral stabilization of the pelvis is lacking. The result is a *Trendelenburg* limp, characterized by a lowering of the pelvis on the normal side when the affected limb carries the body weight. This type of limp, common among patients with hemiplegia, may be recognized at a glance by observing the summit of the head when the patient walks. Each time the affected limb is in stance phase, the summit of the head is lowered, which is not the case in the corresponding phase on the normal side. It must be pointed out, however, that hyperextension of the affected knee in stance phase also results in a lowering of the summit of the head, so that a close investigation is required. Often a Trendelenburg limp and hyperextension of the knee occur simultaneously.

The Trendelenburg limp can only be observed if the patient is capable of walking alone and without a cane, because when a cane or other support is used the limp becomes disguised. If walking without a cane is not safe, the behavior of the abductor muscles on weight bearing may be observed in the standing position as the patient shifts his weight over the affected limb. If the hip abductor muscles do not respond, it becomes difficult or impossible for the patient to balance on that limb and some assistance by the examiner is required (Fig. 5-2B).

The *trunk forward* item on the gait analysis form indicates that the patient flexes the hip by inclining the trunk forward in early stance and midstance. Such trunk movement often occurs in conjunction with hyperextension of the knee and with insufficient yield of the calf muscles in midstance.

Progression requires a continuous shift of body weight forward. It may be assumed that the patient inclines the trunk forward to compensate for his inability to advance the body weight in a normal manner.

Late Stance, Normal Gait. This phase, utilized in preparation for the swing-through of the limb, is characterized by flexion of the hip (Fig. 4-1). Electromyographic studies by Close (1964) revealed that the deep hip flexor muscles (iliacus, psoas major) show little or no activity at this time. This would indicate that the superficial hip flexor muscles are mainly responsible for the initiation of hip flexion in preparation for the swing phase.

Late Stance, Hemiplegic Gait. Because the dominance of the basic limb synergies

prevents a combination of calf muscle activity with hip and knee flexion, the proper preparation for the swing-through is lacking. In many patients with hemiplegia the required cessation of activity of hip and knee extensor muscles is absent or too slow to allow flexion of these joints. The calf muscles may persist in their activity throughout stance, but the rapid rise in tension needed for the push-off is missing.

SWING PHASE: NORMAL GAIT

When the behavior of the three weight-bearing joints in stance phase has been observed and recorded, attention is focused on the manner in which the hemiplegic limb is brought forward.

As pointed out above, swing phase is initiated during the last portion of stance when muscular and gravitational forces act to bring about a forward acceleration of the limb. Electromyograms indicate that muscular activity is minimal during most of swing phase, the limb then moving forward mainly by inertia. The dorsiflexor muscles of the ankle (pretibial group, Fig. 4-2) show slight activity throughout swing phase, to prevent a drop foot. Toward the end of swing phase, muscular activity picks up for the purpose of decelerating the limb in preparation for weight bearing.

SWING PHASE, HEMIPLEGIC GAIT

In general, when the extensor synergy does not let go its grip in late stance or does so too slowly, the limb is moved forward in a stiff manner, hip and knee joints fail to flex or flex insufficiently, and the ankle remains in plantar flexion. Those patients who are capable of activating the flexor synergy do so in an exaggerated manner, particularly as far as the hip is concerned. The exaggerated hip flexion is accompanied by belated flexion of the knee and by dorsiflexion of the ankle.

The swing phase items listed on the gait

analysis form will now be discussed briefly.

Ankle. Failure of the dorsiflexor muscles of the ankle to contract during swing phase results in a drop foot and insufficient ground clearance, which is recorded as *toes dragging*. More often than not, the ankle simultaneously *inverts*, and, if markedly so, it may not be safe for the patient to walk without an ankle brace that restricts inversion. *Exaggerated dorsiflexion* occurs in patients who are activating the flexor synergy in an exaggerated way. *Whip* is a term difficult to describe accurately. A rapid back-and-forth movement takes place, probably at the subtalar joints. The ankle appears unstable, but the position of the foot corrects itself prior to weight bearing.

Knee. Failure of the knee to flex normally during swing phase is recorded as *stiff*, or *moderately stiff*, depending upon the degree of tension that persists in the quadriceps muscles during swing phase. *Exaggerated flexion* indicates that the patient uses the total flexor synergy. Actually, the amount of knee flexion that occurs may not exceed that of normal walking, but the onset of knee flexion is delayed, probably because the calf muscles do not provide the proper push-off in late stance. The knee is lifted forward and upward, the leg hangs more or less vertically, and the foot is well above the ground, as if the patient were stepping over an obstacle.

Hip. With the persistence of the extensor synergy, or delayed release of extensor tension, a normal shortening of the limb required for the swing-through is absent and the patient must find other ways to bring the affected limb forward. In order to get toe clearance either a *circumduction* movement of the limb or a *pelvic hike* on the affected side may be utilized. If the hip is held *stiff* (no hip flexion), the patient may nevertheless succeed in advancing the affected limb by tilting the pelvis backward; the gait then resembles that of a patient with an ankylosed hip. A *moderately stiff hip* is a common appearance, necessitating some anteroposterior or lateral pelvic movements. *Exaggerated flexion* of the hip occurs when the patient utilizes the total flexor synergy, as described above.

Occasionally, a patient may drag the affected limb, never advancing it beyond the normal foot. The pelvis stays behind on the affected side and the hip is *externally rotated*, so that the toes point in a lateral direction. Eversion of the ankle may accompany this gait, but such eversion is not caused by spastic evertor muscles but determined by the limb position, possibly in conjunction with a preexisting flat foot.

REFERENCES

BARD, G. Energy expenditure of hemiplegic subjects during walking. *Arch. Phys. Med.* 44:368, 1963.

BARD, G., and RALSTON, H. J. Measurement of energy expenditure during ambulation, with special reference to evaluation of assistive devices. *Arch. Phys. Med.* 40:415, 1959.

CLOSE, J. R. *Motor Function in the Lower Extremity, Analysis by Electronic Instrumentation.* Springfield, Ill., Thomas, 1964, p. 127.

EBERHART, H. D., INMAN, V. T., and ASSOCIATES. *Fundamental Studies of Human Locomotion and Other Information Relating to Design of Artificial Limbs.* Report to National Research Council, Univ. of Calif. College of Engineering, Berkeley, 1947. Vol. I, Sections 3 and 4.

HIRSCHBERG, G. G., and NATHANSON, K. Electromyographic recording of muscular activity in normal and spastic gaits. *Arch. Phys. Med.* 33:217, 1952.

Under normal circumstances, walking is an automatic activity, that is, no attention is given to the details of its execution. The sole responsibility of the will is to give a walking command, and the central nervous system centers responsible for human locomotion patterns take over. When the nervous system through disease or injury has undergone "evolution in reverse" (Jackson, 1884), these patterns are no longer accessible and the individual must adapt to circumstances and utilize patterns still available—in the case of patients with hemiplegia, the basic limb synergies. As discussed in Chapter 4, muscular associations characteristic of the basic limb synergies differ considerably from the requirements of normal locomotion.

During the period when the basic limb synergies dominate the motor behavior, the problem of ambulation is solved by individual patients in different ways. It is the individual's choice of compensation as well as the severity of the involvement that determines the ambulation pattern. Once a specific pattern has evolved, it is likely to become firmly established, hence difficult to change.

Many patients are potentially capable of becoming good or at least fair walkers; yet, a poor pattern, once established, may stubbornly resist correction. During the early period following the onset of hemiplegia, it would therefore seem advisable to concentrate on *preparation* for walking while postponing actual walking, or extensive walking, for some time, in order to avoid the establishment of a poor gait pattern. This does not mean that all weight bearing should be avoided; a number of weight-bearing exercises and activities may and should be practiced as soon as feasible.

Preparation for walking will be discussed in some detail below, while less time will be devoted to what may be called "conventional gait training." The

Walking Preparation and Gait Training

111

author contends that in many instances this approach will pay dividends in terms of final outcome. In the case of severely involved patients whose chances to progress beyond the synergy stages appear to be slim, a compromise has to be reached.

Preparation for walking should include (1) training in trunk balance, sitting, and standing; (2) modification of motor responses of the limbs to obtain muscular associations resembling those required for normal walking; and (3) training of alternate responses of antagonistic muscles, such as flexors and extensors, to promote a rapid release in tension of muscle groups following their activation. The three types of training will be discussed under three headings, but they are not separate entities. Thus, modification of motor responses of the limbs and training of alternate contractions of agonistic and antagonistic muscle groups takes place simultaneously. In addition, and as an integral part of the training program, attention is given to the strengthening of weak muscles, because weakness is often concomitant with other muscular deficiencies in patients with hemiplegia.

TRUNK BALANCE

The upright posture—whether sitting, standing, or walking—requires the proper functioning of a number of central balancing mechanisms. Afferent impulses of widespread origins, including signals from the periphery, play important roles in eliciting and guiding responses, while efferent pathways carry messages to the muscles for the execution of the balancing act. Damage to any one of the central mechanisms or interruption anywhere along the sensory or motor pathways subserving the central mechanisms might result in deficient balance.

A discussion of the neurophysiology of normal balance and of the neuropathology responsible for impairment in balance in patients with hemiplegia lies outside the scope of this manual. Students are advised to consult other sources for elucidation of this complex subject matter.

TRUNK LISTING IN SITTING

Success in maintaining standing balance cannot be expected unless and until the patient can balance the trunk in the sitting position without relying on back or side support. Some patients with hemiplegia have good sitting balance at an early date, others have a tendency to list toward the side, almost invariably toward the affected side, when they sit unsupported (Fig. 3-2). Therapeutic procedures to improve trunk balance in sitting are described and illustrated in Chapter 3.

Beevor's Observations

The tendency of patients with hemiplegia to list toward the affected body side was discussed at great length by Beevor, who investigated unresisted and resisted side motions of the trunk, testing shortening and lengthening contractions of trunk muscles on both sides of the midline (Beevor, 1909). The investigations were carried out in both the sitting and supine positions. Beevor concluded that a patient with, for example, left-sided involvement who displayed the listing phenomenon had difficulty in, or was incapable of, controlling his trunk whenever the motion took place to the left of the midline, regardless of which muscles were needed for control. Motions to the right of the midline were well under control, as were movements requiring simultaneous action of trunk muscles on both sides of the midline, as in flexion and extension of the vertebral column.

Deficiency of Perception

More recent studies by Bruell and associates (1956, 1957), and by Birch and associates (1960, 1961) suggest that the listing phenomenon of patients with hemiplegia may be related to a deficiency in the perception of spatial relationships. According to Birch and associates, patients with left-sided involvement tend to make errors of judgment of the vertical and horizontal in a counterclockwise direction, and, by adjusting their body posture to what they perceive as vertical, they tend to deviate toward the left. The implications for ambulation in terms of prevention of falls for these patients is stressed.

If the perception of verticality is imperfect, attempts should be made to help the patient gain a better appreciation of spatial relations. It may be assumed that, in spite of possible permanent damage, the patient may improve his judgment by utilizing, to the best possible extent, those mechanisms that remain functional. For this purpose, reinforcement of afferent impulses from receptors for position sense, kinesthesis, pressure, light touch, and so on, as well as emphasis on specific visual clues, have been found useful. A light touch by the normal hand on a horizontal or vertical stationary object, a temporary raise under the buttock on one side or the other, and repetitive head and trunk movements are examples of methods of approach.

Trunk movements, whether passive or active, assisted or resisted, are considered useful in several respects. Afferent impulses thus evoked contribute not only to coordination of trunk movements and thus to balance, but also produce reflex effects on the limbs (see Chapter 3). Rhythmic rotary movements of the trunk should be given special attention; such movements are required in walking and are essential for proper coordination of arm and leg movements in walking.

The arm position illustrated in Figures 3-3 and 3-4 is convenient for trunk movements forward and backward and for trunk rotation movements. The physical therapist sits facing the patient and guides the movements until the patient becomes confident enough to continue unaided. For lateral trunk bending, the patient's arm should be unrestricted so that he can reach for objects of proper height placed on the floor. Care must be exercised because reaching toward the floor may cause loss of balance.

Trunk balance and trunk rotation exercises in standing belong in an advanced stage and will be discussed later.

MODIFICATION OF MOTOR RESPONSES OF THE LOWER LIMB

INDICATIONS FOR SPECIAL TRAINING PROCEDURES

Modification of motor responses is indicated when the basic limb synergies dominate motor acts and thus prevent the return of normal gait patterns. In the most severe cases, however, attempts to break up the synergies may never succeed and will have to be given up; more modest ambulation aims should then be set. On the other hand, when the involvement is mild, modification of motor responses may not be necessary because the synergies soon lose their grip, and spontaneous return of normal or near normal gait patterns may then be expected. The largest number of patients, however, fall between the two extremes of the severely involved and the mildly involved, and for this group modification of synergy responses is indicated.

REQUIREMENTS FOR THE EARLY STANCE PHASE

During normal level walking the following muscle groups show electrical activities in the early stance phase: the dorsiflexors of the ankle, the extensors of the knee, the extensors of the hip, and the abductors of the hip (see Fig. 4-2). In contradistinction, the extensor synergy, which is activated on weight bearing in patients with hemiplegia, combines hip and knee extension with plantar flexion of the ankle and adduction of the hip. If somewhat more normal muscle associations are to be established, *the dorsiflexors of the ankle and the abductors of the hip must be activated and induced to associate themselves with the extensors of hip and knee, and this association must materialize in the early stance phase.*

ACTIVATION OF THE DORSIFLEXOR MUSCLES OF THE ANKLE

A patient may be incapable under any circumstances, regardless of movement combinations, of activating the dorsiflexor muscles of the ankle voluntarily. In this case, the first approach is to elicit a reflex response in this muscle group as a component part of the total flexor synergy, a later objective being to cause these muscles to act together with the extensor muscles of hip and knee.

Reflex Response

A well-known procedure for eliciting response in the dorsiflexor muscles of the ankle is to resist hip flexion when the latter motion is under voluntary control. But when the patient has no control of hip flexion, passive plantar flexion of the toes is administered, and this manipulation usually elicits a mass flexor response, which includes dorsiflexion of the ankle. The response is known as Bechterev's reflex, after the Russian neurologist. Some-

times it is referred to as the Marie-Foix reflex, after the French neurologist Pierre Marie and his associate, C. Foix. The reflex is elicited with the patient in the supine position, knees extended. The limb position and the physical therapist's grip around the patient's toes, when voluntary effort is added, are illustrated in Figure 5-1.

Introducing Voluntary Effort

When reflex contractions of the dorsiflexor muscles of the ankle have been evoked a number of times, the patient's voluntary effort is superimposed on the reflex contraction. The proper timing of the voluntary effort with the reflex contraction is of utmost importance because the reflex tension may fade out rather rapidly.

When a good response is obtained, the physical therapist resists the total flexor movement by pressing against the dorsum of the patient's foot, while simultaneously giving the emphatic command, "Don't let me pull your foot down." If the ankle response is poor, manual resistance may also be given to hip flexion, but ankle resistance alone is preferred because this is the movement to be emphasized.

Reinforcement of Voluntary Effort

The next step in training the dorsiflexor muscles of the ankle is to have the patient actively attempt to initiate the movement without the use of reflex elicitation. The supine or the sitting position may now be

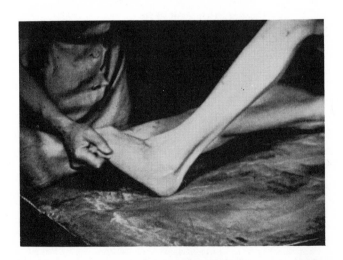

FIGURE 5-1. Bechterev's reflex is elicited by passive plantar flexion of the toes. Voluntary impulses are superimposed on the reflex effect (see text). (Frame of a motion picture.)

utilized. The physical therapist places one of his hands on the patient's thigh on the involved side just above the knee, pressing down slightly; should the hip flexor muscles contract together with the pretibial muscles, the pressure is increased. Even though the hip flexor muscles may become active, hip flexion must not be permitted at this time because the objective is to obtain a more isolated response at the ankle. Local facilitatory measures, such as vigorous rubbing of the skin over the bellies of the pretibial muscles or percussion of their tendons as these pass the ankle joint, often prove effective. A lengthening or isometric contraction is first required ("Don't let me pull your foot down"), then a shortening contraction ("Now pull your foot up again"). If the patient is supine, the procedure is repeated in positions incorporating less and less flexion of hip and knee, so that the extended position is gradually approached.

Dorsiflexion of the Ankle in Standing

When a patient can voluntarily dorsiflex the ankle sitting on an ordinary chair, he changes to a higher chair, sitting on its edge only; then he stands leaning his buttocks against a table of proper height, then stands with his back to a wall, and finally stands without support with the affected foot forward in a position of a short step. The amount of stabilization and local facilitation offered by the physical therapist is gradually diminished as better voluntary control is gained.

Dorsiflexion with Eversion

Throughout the training of the pretibial muscles, attention is paid to proper positioning of the ankle and to the placement of the resisting hand for the purpose of causing the long toe extensor muscles and, eventually, the peroneal muscles to participate. The physical therapist's resisting hand gradually moves in a lateral direction where it is in a good position to apply resistance to eversion, should there be a favorable response. The therapist may also try a sudden inversion movement of the patient's foot to evoke a stretch reflex in the peroneal muscles; if the tension thus created is picked up by resistance, the duration of the muscle tension may be prolonged. Percussion or stroking over the evertor muscles may also be effective, and sometimes a vigorous rubbing on the lateral aspect of the foot brings results.

When these procedures are first applied it is of no avail to ask the patient to evert the foot, because this would only detract from his effort to pull the foot up, an effort that must be sustained. It is the physical therapist's task to employ facilitatory measures to shunt the impulses that are set up by the patient's effort into slightly different pathways—in this case, to cause the impulses to spread to the lateral muscles. Not until the activation of these muscles has become a reality should the concept of holding the foot in an everted position against the physical therapist's inversion motion be brought to the patient's attention. The terms *inversion* and *eversion* should be avoided. Instead, commands may be used such as "Hold your foot steady, Don't let me turn your foot in," and later, "Now turn your foot out again."

The above procedure follows the general principles of (1) having the patient attempt only those motions that are, at least in part, under voluntary control, or that may be expected to succeed in the near future; (2) modifying the movements that have been obtained to include other components; and (3) requiring isometric or lengthening contractions before shortening contractions.

ACTIVATION OF THE ABDUCTOR MUSCLES OF THE HIP

The Trendelenburg limp, common among patients with hemiplegia, is related to the firm association of the components of the extensor synergy, to the exclusion of other muscular combinations. Because the abductor muscles belong to the flexor synergy, they refuse to act upon weight bearing, which they normally do, and the result is loss of lateral stabilization of the pelvis on the affected side (Fig. 5-2).

The approach to this situation is similar to the one outlined for the dorsiflexor muscles of the ankle:

1. If voluntary control is not present in any position or movement combination, a contraction is elicited reflexly.
2. The patient superimposes his voluntary effort on the reflex contraction.
3. Local facilitatory measures are introduced to reinforce the patient's voluntary effort.
4. Attempts are made to cause the muscle groups that have been activated to respond in the desired situation—in this case, in early stance phase, continuing into midstance.

Reflex Response

Raimiste's phenomenon, discussed in Chapter 1, is utilized to evoke a reflex contraction in the abductor muscles of the hip and to facilitate and strengthen the contraction of these muscles. In using the Rai-

miste's phenomenon, it will be found that adduction is more readily evoked than abduction, probably because hip and knee joints are extended in the supine position, and because adduction and extension are linked in the extensor synergy. However, reflex abduction of the affected limb can usually be elicited if resistance on the normal side is strong and sustained. The reflex response always lags behind the stimulus by means of which it is evoked.

Figure 5-3*A* and *B* shows the adduction response and Figure 5-3*C* the abduction response of a patient with left-sided hemiparesis. The abduction response is almost full range, but strong sustained effort on the normal side was required. The phenomena as originally described by Raimiste are evoked by strong *isometric* contractions of the abductor or adductor muscles on the normal side. In the illustrations, resisted *shortening* contractions have been used.

For training purposes, the physical therapist stands at the foot of the table, which enables him to give bilateral resistance to abduction and adduction.

Alternate Abduction and Adduction

It is suggested that resistance to abduction on the normal side be given repeatedly until some contralateral response is noticed. Thereafter, abduction and adduction responses are evoked alternately and this method appears to reinforce both responses, provided the proper timing is

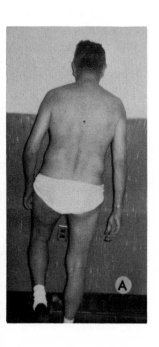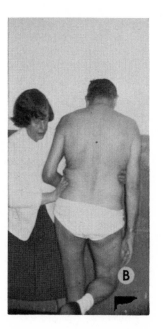

FIGURE 5-2. Trendelenburg sign in 53-year-old patient with left-sided hemiparesis of 7 months' duration, following an intracranial hemorrhage and surgery. The patient walked with a marked Trendelenburg limp. *A.* Balance on the unaffected limb is excellent. The abductor muscles on the right side stabilize the pelvis. The left side of the pelvis is higher than the right. *B.* Patient is assisted to shift the body weight over to the affected limb. He cannot balance unaided. The right side of the pelvis becomes lowered because of loss of the stabilizing action of the abductor muscles on the left side.

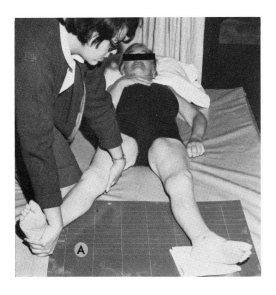

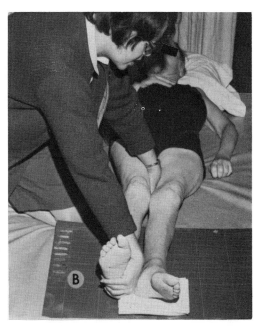

observed. The physical therapist's hands must move from one side of the ankles to the other in order to take advantage of the brief interval during which each successive motion is facilitated. Possibly, this facilitation is a manifestation of "successive induction" described by Sherrington, a mechanism that enhances the contraction of agonistic and antagonistic muscles in rhythmic succession in spinal animals (Sherrington, 1947, p. 209). It is understood that the patient's voluntary effort is superimposed on the reflex contraction and that also unilateral abduction is practiced when this becomes possible.

Success in directing voluntary impulses to the abductor muscles on the affected side in the supine position, however, is only the beginning. The abductor muscles must then be strengthened to enable them, mechanically, to perform their weight-bearing function. Most importantly, these muscles must become associated with the extensor muscles of hip and knee during the early stance phase.

FIGURE 5-3. Raimiste's phenomena in patient with left-sided hemiparesis. *A.* The patient's both lower limbs have been passively abducted, and the physical therapist has placed her hands on the medial side of the patient's normal limb. Thereafter, the patient is asked to adduct the normal limb against resistance. *B.* Adduction of the normal limb has been completed by voluntary effort; simultaneously, the affected limb has adducted reflexly. *C.* When the limbs are in the adducted position, as in Figure 5-3*B*, the physical therapist switches her hands from the inside to the outside of the patient's normal limb and asks the patient to abduct this limb against resistance. If the resistance is sufficiently strong, the affected limb will abduct reflexly, as it has done in *C.*

Hip Abduction, Side-lying Position

The patient lies on his unaffected side with the hip and knee on that side partially flexed. The physical therapist stands behind the patient, lifts the affected limb

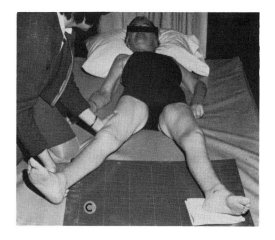

into partial abduction, then proceeds to stimulate the gluteal muscles by means of vigorous gross percussion. Such percussion or "beating" is performed as a wrist movement with one hand, fist closed. The purpose of this stimulation must first be explained to the patient. Although one patient may be told that he is going to get "a good beating" in order to "wake up those lazy muscles," another patient will have to be informed in different words.

Immediately following the "beating" of the abductor muscles, the command "Hold, don't let your leg fall down" is given; simultaneously the physical therapist momentarily allows the limb to fall a very short distance if the patient is unable to comply with the command; then the procedure is repeated. This method aims at building up a reflex tension in the abductor muscles, which tension, if augmented by a voluntary effort, may result in a muscular contraction strong enough to hold the limb in the desired position, or at least to slow its downward movement.

Bilateral Action of the Hip-Abductor Muscles in Standing.

This is an advanced training procedure which consists of swinging first the affected then the unaffected limb to the side (into abduction) and which involves momentary weight bearing on one leg at a time. It is discussed here because it belongs to the sequence employed in evoking responses in the abductor muscles of the hip for the prevention or correction of a Trendelenburg limp. It must be understood, however, that it must be preceded by nonweight-bearing training and by preliminary weight-bearing practice.

Normally, when one leg is taken off the ground, as in Figure 5-2A, the abductor muscles on the stance side automatically contract for lateral stabilization of the pelvis. The same occurs if the off-ground limb is raised laterally into abduction, which consequently results in *bilateral* acti-

vation of the hip-abductor muscles. In the case of a patient with hemiplegia, it is hoped that, owing to the muscular contraction on the normal side, the abductor muscles on the affected side may become facilitated. However, it is not known to what extent, if any, the Raimiste's phenomenon applies to the standing as well as to the supine position.

The patient stands facing a firm object, such as parallel bars, and uses his normal hand to support himself while the therapist stands behind him to guide and stabilize as needed. Assuming that the left side is the affected one, the patient first shifts his weight over the right limb and swings his left one toward the side. This can be done within small range by a pelvic movement, even if the abductor muscles proper do not respond.

With the physical therapist's assistance, the body weight is next shifted toward the left. Pressure downward on the left iliac crest and upward on the right side of the pelvis, if given with sufficient force, will prevent a sagging of the pelvis on the right side. Simultaneously, the patient is encouraged to raise the right limb into abduction. The patient hesitates to do this because he has little or no balancing ability on the left leg. Adequate assistance by the physical therapist is essential at this time. Local stimulation ("beating") of the hip-abductor muscles on the left side before and during the weight shift is also indicated if it can be managed without endangering the patient's balance.

Unilateral Action of the Hip-Abductor Muscles in Standing

This is the last and the most demanding activity in the sequence of procedures designed to activate and strengthen the hip-abductor muscles on the affected side. The exercise has little chance of success unless the abductor muscles are capable of associating with the extensor muscles of hip and knee, that is, until the influence of the basic limb synergies has vanished, or practically vanished. It is employed to emphasize and strengthen a muscle combination already feasible.

In the standing position, the patient is instructed to elevate ("hike") the pelvis on the unaffected side, enough to lift the foot on that side off the ground. This, of course, necessitates a strong contraction of the hip-abductor muscles on the opposite side. Few individuals with normal neuromuscular control (except physical therapists!) are aware that such hip-hiking is accomplished mainly by muscles on the opposite side. It would serve no good purpose and would only confuse the issue to point out to the patient which muscle group is expected to contract. The patient's attention should be focused on "hip-hiking" on the unaffected side.

At the beginning, the patient uses his normal hand for support and the physical therapist assists to emphasize the pelvic movement and to steady the patient. The hip-hiking movement performed on alternate sides represents a transition to the actual walking situation and may later be repeated during walking. The patient is encouraged to "grow tall" on each step and to use a smooth walking rhythm; a suitable cadence may be provided by the therapist's voice. The use of a cane during this type of training is not recommended because it interferes with the walking rhythm. Furthermore, leaning heavily on a cane relieves the abductor muscles on the opposite side of their weight-bearing function, hence nothing is gained in terms of strengthening the abductor muscles.

If the method of activating the hip abductor muscles described above are successful and these muscles respond with sufficient strength, lateral stabilization of the pelvis has been reestablished. However, elimination of the Trendelenburg limp cannot be expected to succeed in every patient with hemiplegia, and good judgment must be exercised to determine how long this particular aspect of training

should continue. If the Trendelenburg limp persists, the patient should be encouraged to use a cane, at least when walking outdoors, to minimize the limp and guard the abductor muscles on the affected side from being over-stretched.

ALTERNATE RESPONSES OF ANTAGONISTIC MUSCLES

KNEE FLEXORS AND KNEE EXTENSORS

It has previously been pointed out that in patients with hemiplegia the extensor synergy predominates in the lower, and the flexor synergy in the upper limb. As a result, extensor responses can usually be evoked in the lower limb without too much difficulty, except in the early stage of flaccidity which follows a cerebral vascular accident, and in those cases where flaccidity persists for longer periods of time.

However, once an extensor response has been obtained, it is likely to continue too long to comply with changing requirements during postural sway in standing and during walking. The inability of spastic muscles to release their tension rapidly and at the proper time adversely affects all coordinated activities and markedly impairs locomotion. A rapid fall in tension in the knee extensor muscles following their peak contraction shortly after heel contact, as required in normal walking, cannot be duplicated by these muscles. The failure of the quadriceps muscles to cease contracting at the proper time is one of the major causes of disturbance of the walking pattern in patients with hemiplegia.

The training methods to be chosen depend to a great extent on the flaccidity-spasticity status of the patient. During the flaccid state the quadriceps muscles must be stimulated; during spasticity, inhibited. In both instances, however, *alternating action of knee flexor and knee extensor muscles is stressed* in order to decrease the duration of contraction of opposing sets of muscles.

Special emphasis on the training of the knee flexor muscles is usually indicated, and this may be done in supine, sitting, "half-prone," and standing positions. More or less isolated responses of the knee flexor muscles are desirable, but regardless of success in this respect, alternate activation of flexor and extensor muscles is essential.

Supine Position

In certain patients, the supine position in itself suffices to cause a fixation of the knee in extension (labyrinthine influence), which prevents voluntary flexion of the knee. In such cases, local stimulation of the tendons of the hamstring muscles, or manipulation of the soft tissue on the posterior side of the thigh, sometimes is sufficient to release tension in the quadriceps muscles. With the knee joint no longer "locked" in extension but held in slight flexion, the patient may now be able to initiate the flexor synergy, which he could not do previously. A modification of the flexor synergy is then attempted for the purpose of limiting hip flexion and increasing range of motion at the knee. While the patient pulls his knee up toward the chest, the physical therapist holds the foot down so that the sole slides on the horizontal surface. This movement is repeated several times. The sensation thus evoked is emphasized: "Do you feel the sole of the foot sliding on the table?" "Feel it again." And after a few trials: "Now keep touching the table and slide your foot back yourself." Alternate knee flexion and extension movements in small range are then attempted without permitting the sole of the foot to leave the table. This movement requires partial inhibition of the hip flexor muscles and active contraction of the knee flexor muscles, which contraction is reinforced by resistance. Speed is increased when feasible.

Sitting Position

If the knee flexor muscles cannot be induced to contract in the supine position, activation of these muscles practically always succeeds in the sitting position. The patient sits on a firm chair and places his foot forward on the floor, the heel touching and the knee short of full extension. He then slides the foot backward, touching the floor with the heel and then with the ball of the foot, as the foot slides underneath the chair and the knee flexes to an acute angle. This movement is first performed several times on the normal side, then attempted on the affected side. At the onset, the physical therapist may have to assist the backward sliding movement of the foot directly, or aid by lifting the lower portion of the patient's thigh just enough to reduce friction of the patient's foot on the floor. The lifting is accomplished by a grip from below, just above the knee; this grip also permits palpation and manipulation of the tendons of the knee flexor muscles.

The sitting position offers several advantages for the activation of the biceps femoris and the semitendinosus and the semimembranosus muscles. First, knee flexion is facilitated because the hip and knee are flexed, and the two-joint knee flexor muscles are relatively elongated. Second, the hip angle changes very little during the motion so that the patient experiences the sensation of a more or less isolated knee motion. Third, the sliding of the foot on the floor serves as a guide for the motion. Fourth, the position lends itself well for an additional type of facilitation, which will now be described.

It is assumed that the patient, seated on a chair and keeping the soles of both feet flat on the floor, has learned to incline the trunk forward while supporting the elbow on the affected side with the normal hand, as seen in Figure 3-3. By palpating the tendons at the knee the physical therapist may ascertain whether or not the knee flexor muscles have been activated when the patient inclines the trunk forward. This is almost always the case. This response of the hamstring muscles may be thought of primarily as an automatic reaction for the purpose of balancing the trunk at the hip. It appears to be easier to evoke a contraction of these muscles when they are needed as hip extensors than when knee flexion is willed. Note also that these two-joint muscles become further elongated as the trunk inclines forward, and this too might facilitate their contraction.

The effect of forward inclination of the trunk on the patient's ability to flex the knee by sliding the foot backward is seen in Figure 5-4. When the knee cannot be flexed beyond 90 degrees (Fig. 5-4A), the patient learns to synchronize a forward inclination of the trunk with an effort to slide the foot backward, and additional knee flexion may result (Fig. 5-4B). The psychological effect of this success is often remarkable as the patient experiences the sensation of moving the foot backward by voluntary effort. After completion of knee flexion, the patient leans against the back of the chair and extends the knee to the starting position. When control has improved, alternation between knee flexion and knee extension in increasingly rapid succession and in varying joint ranges begins, with or without accompanying trunk movements.

"Half-prone" Position

The patient leans over a table so that the trunk is supported on the table and the hips are flexed over the edge of the table. The patient stabilizes himself with the normal hand and the physical therapist furnishes additional stabilization when needed. In this half-prone position isolated

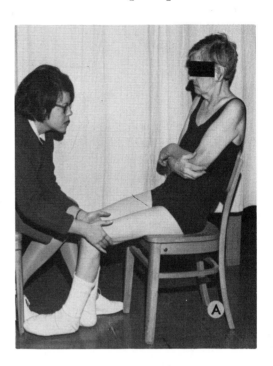

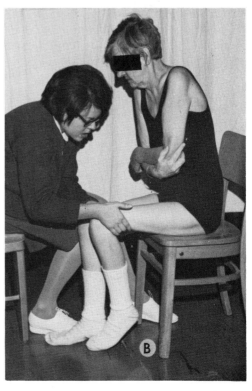

FIGURE 5-4. Activation of knee flexor muscles in patient with left-sided hemiparesis. *A.* Patient is unable to slide the foot backward even thought the therapist lessens the heel pressure on the floor by a grip around the thigh near the knee. *B.* As the patient inclines the trunk forward, the hamstring muscles are elongated and activated as hip extensors. The background tension thus created enables the patient to flex the affected knee to an acute angle by sliding the foot backward.

knee flexion is attempted by the patient and resistance is given as soon as a response is obtained. Stimulation by percussion or vigorous stroking over portions of the muscles of the posterior thigh may also be required to get the movement started. For alternate responses, resistance is given to extension of the knee.

Standing Position

The half-prone position is gradually modified to a standing position with the patient facing and leaning against a higher object, such as a chest of drawers. Eventually, the patient stands fully erect using hand support only. When in this position flexion of the affected limb can be performed while the hip on the affected side is kept extended, it is a sign that the hemiplegic limb synergies no longer influence the patient's movements.

PREDOMINANCE OF FLEXION IN THE LOWER LIMB

In rather unusual cases, the flexor synergy dominates the motor behavior of the lower limb, sometimes to the extent that the patient is unable to lower the limb to the table in the supine position or to the floor in standing. The patient in Figure 5-5 is an example. Figure 5-5A shows the usual posture of the limb in the supine position. If an attempt was made to straighten out the limb passively, flexor tension increased and the limb withdrew. However, flexor tension could be released if, without traction on the affected limb, both limbs were raised somewhat by the physical therapist who then carried out rhythmic side-to-side movements of both limbs within small range. Gradually, the affected limb assumed a more normal position (Fig. 5-5B) and remained extended when the limbs were gently lowered to the supporting surface.

A return to a flexed position, however, was observed if the patient became excited, and the flexor synergy was regularly evoked as an associated movement if the patient made a muscular effort on the unaffected side, as in Figure 5-5D.

If the patient was assisted to the standing position, his hip and knee remained flexed on the affected side and he was unable to lower the foot to the ground. Two therapists were required to support the patient and to place his foot on a 2-inch-high wooden board; this was accomplished by hand pressure against the sole of the foot and friction over the quadriceps muscles. The foot was stabilized on the board and pressure was applied on the knee (Fig. 5-6A). After some practice the support under the foot on the affected side was lowered, and a reasonably good standing position with the affected limb carrying some of the body weight was achieved (Fig. 5-6B). But it was a precarious position because if the patient was allowed to shift his weight back over the other limb, the affected foot tended to lose its contact with the board and the limb went into extreme adduction (Fig. 5-6C), a limb position quite unsuitable for locomotion. However, a withdrawal of the limb to its earlier flexed position did not occur—that is, muscular tension had been shifted from flexor to extensor muscles.

It would seem at first as though ambulation were not feasible when the adduction component of the extensor synergy is so strong that the involved limb crosses in front of the normal limb and when this movement cannot be modified by the patient. However, the author's experience indicates that adduction may become partially inhibited if the ankle is controlled by a brace that prevents plantar flexion and inversion. Only limited success in ambulation may be expected of a patient who exhibits strong involuntary movement synergies and severe spasticity, as did the patient in Figures 5-5 and 5-6.

STANDING AND WALKING

KNEE STABILITY IN
STANDING AND WALKING

In general, weight bearing on the affected limb is likely to evoke a response of the quadriceps muscles, but satisfactory knee stability does not always materialize. The knee may give way and cause a fall, or the knee may snap into hyperextension, a safe but undesirable position. In either case, training approaches are similar, inasmuch as *the patient must learn momentarily to support weight on a slightly flexed knee.*

Standing Knee Bends. As a safety measure, the physical therapist or an assistant stands behind the patient, supporting his trunk on both sides of the chest. The patient is guided in shifting his weight toward the affected side with both knees slightly flexed. Thereafter, the knees are flexed an additional 10 to 20 degrees, then extended, but not hyperextended. A satisfactory response of the knee extensor muscles will probably be evoked also on the affected side. But should such response fail to appear, the physical therapist is in a position to prevent a fall. When the patient becomes more confident, support may be withdrawn. However, if the patient fails to distribute weight equally on the two legs, guidance and support is resumed.

"Marking Time," Knees Slightly Flexed. This requires momentary full weight bearing on the affected limb while the other limb is raised off the ground. It is not as difficult to accomplish as it may seem at first because the antigravity muscles usually respond under circumstances of forced weight bearing.

Forward Progression, Knees Slightly Flexed. The therapist supports the patient on the unaffected side to permit firm and secure control of weight shift and to prevent a fall. When walking with flexed knees is first attempted, the therapist walks with the patient, keeps his own knees flexed, takes short steps, and encourages the patient to do the same. The walk actually becomes a "shuffling along," the entire sole of the foot being placed on the ground while hips and knees remain slightly flexed. A moderate amount of forward inclination of the trunk is permitted because it reduces the strain on the knee extensor muscles. At a later date, the inclination of the trunk may be increased and decreased at regular intervals—for example, on every fourth step—so that the knee extensor muscles may learn to adjust their activity to changing requirements. It has been observed that patients with hemiplegia, when walking with flexed knees next to an instructor, are capable of a comparatively rapid succession of steps without being restrained by spasticity in the quadriceps muscles.

PREPARATION FOR "SWING-THROUGH" IN WALKING

The purpose of this activity is to obtain a rapid release of tension in the quadriceps muscles and sufficient knee flexion to allow the affected limb to swing through freely in walking. It has some resemblance to a bicycling movement, as it goes around and around; it is perhaps best compared to a horse's pawing as the animal scrapes the ground with the forefoot.

The patient uses hand support to minimize balancing difficulties and performs with the normal then with the affected limb. At first the physical therapist may have to assist in keeping the ball of the foot in contact with the ground on the affected side during the backward scraping movement. The affected limb performs four to six times before a change is made to the other side. Eventually, a walking rhythm—once right, once left—is attempted.

The above movement requires simultaneous use of knee flexor and hip extensor muscles and is therefore difficult as long as the basic limb synergies are influential. If this is the case, the patient may first practice a slow movement of hip-knee flexion with emphasis on knee flexion in the following manner. The contact of the foot with the ground is maintained during the backward movement, and when the foot is taken off the ground, the foot is made to follow the inner side of the normal leg, sliding up toward the knee. This requires a considerable amount of activity of the knee flexor muscles and a reciprocal decrease in tension of the knee extensor muscles.

TRUNK ROTATION WITH ARM SWINGING

This exercise is designed to mobilize the trunk to permit participation by the trunk and free swinging of the arms, first in standing, then in walking. As the trunk rotates, the body weight is shifted from one side to the other; the arms tend to participate automatically, probably influenced by afferent impulses originating in the lumbar region.

It is well known that patients with hemiplegia tend to walk without much trunk rotation and, if spasticity is present in the upper limb, with the elbow flexed and the shoulder immobilized. Although full return to normal arm swinging cannot be expected as long as spasticity persists, the benefit that may be derived from training is not to be ignored.

Trunk rotation in the sitting position has been described in Chapter 3, where it was suggested that the patient's arms be folded in front of the chest. In the standing position, the arms should hang freely from the shoulders and an effort should be made to "wrap" them around the body as the trunk rotates from side to side. This movement is part of advanced training and prerequisite is a fairly good general balance. However, it also aids in developing balance, and if proper precautions are taken it may be used also for less advanced patients.

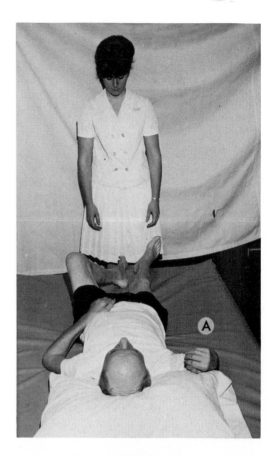

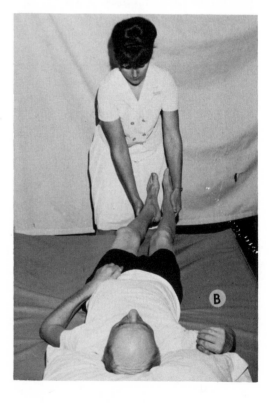

FIGURE 5-5. A 65-year-old patient with left-sided hemiparesis, 4 months following a cerebral vascular accident, exhibiting marked predominance of the flexor synergy of the lower limb. *A.* Flexor tension persists in the supine position and is increased if an attempt is made to extend the limb passively. *B.* If the limbs are gently elevated from the supporting surface without traction on the left limb, and small swinging movements of the limbs from side to side are performed, flexor tension subsides. *C.* Following release of flexor tension, the limb temporarily remains extended. The therapist prepares to resist elbow flexion on the right side. *D.* Resistance to elbow flexion evokes a vigorous associated movement of the affected limb. All components of the flexor synergy appear in full range.

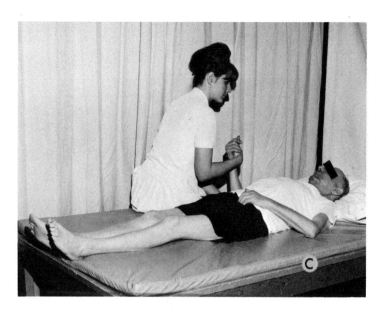

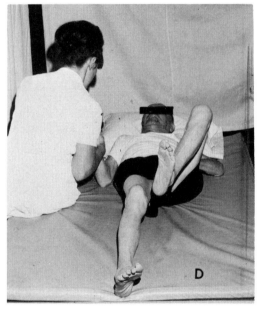

As the trunk rotates to the left, the left arm swings behind the body until the dorsum of the hand reaches the gluteal region; simultaneously, the right arm swings in front of the body, the palm of the hand reaching toward the left side of the body in the region of the greater trochanter. This describes the movement as performed by a normal individual; for the patient with hemiplegia a less perfect movement is to be expected. The arms should be "wrapped" around the body as a result of the trunk movement, not by forceful effort by the patient. The therapist may stand behind the patient, aiding the movements of the arms without forcing them, also being ready to support the patient should he lose his balance.

The next step is slow walking with exaggerated trunk rotation. The arm movements are somewhat modified—the entire "wrap-around" is not attempted. It is understood that when the left foot steps forward the trunk rotates toward the left and the right arm swings forward and across the body, but to avoid confusion no mention is made to the patient of right and left. He is simply told to start walking. As he does so, he is assisted to get the arms moving in the right directions. The rhythm must not be sacrificed even though trunk and arm movements may not be perfect. Manual movement corrections are avoided as these may increase spasticity and frighten the patient and may even throw him off balance.

AUTOMATIC GAIT

A number of nonweight-bearing standing and walking exercises have been outlined, all designed to prepare the patient for an acceptable automatic gait. There are reasons to believe that a favorable neuro-physiological background for the return of a relatively normal gait pattern is provided when the patient has gained control of some of the muscular combinations that are characteristic of normal walking. If the patient's involvement is too severe to expect a lessening of the influence of the basic limb synergies, walking preparation prior to weight bearing may at least aid him in acquiring a relatively safe type of locomotion and may enable him to compensate for his disability in the least objectionable manner.

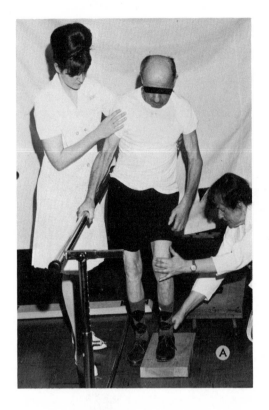

FIGURE 5-6. The patient seen in Figure 5-5 has been assisted to the standing position by two physical therapists. The total flexor synergy first appeared and the foot remained high above the floor. *A.* An extensor response has been evoked, and the patient's body weight has been shifted in part toward the affected foot, which is stabilized on a 2-inch wooden board (see text). *B.* Following some training, a reasonably good standing position has been achieved. *C.* When the weight is shifted toward the normal side, the affected limb assumes a "scissor" posture in front of the other limb.

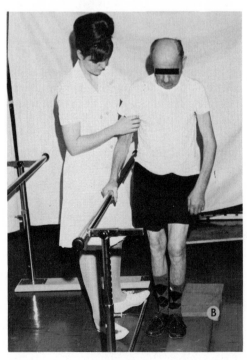

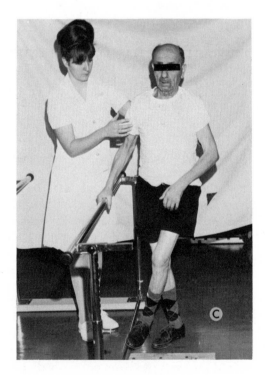

ASSISTED WALKING

A good way of providing safety for the patient when he first walks outside of the parallel bars is for the physical therapist to walk along the patient's unaffected side while grasping the patient's both hands in such a manner that the arms of the two individuals cross each other. This kind of support is helpful for controlling the patient's weight transfer from one limb to the other, for practicing variations in walking cadence and equalization of steps, and so on. If it seems desirable to draw the attention of the patient away from his walking problems, and it often is, the physical therapist may start a conversation unrelated to walking without interrupting the pace. Throughout, instructor and pupil walk in step because the instructor's rhythm has a beneficial effect on the patient's gait. The cadence, of course, must be kept within the patient's capabilities.

WALKING INSTRUCTIONS

When the patient begins to walk, the physical therapist assists and encourages but keeps instructions at a minimum. Too many corrections may annoy the patient, and the effort he would expend in trying to follow instructions might cause an increase in spasticity and interfere with walking rhythm. If suggestions are given, not more than one should be given at a time. For example, attention may be focused on proper weight shift toward the affected side, on preventing hyperextension of the knee, or on touching the ground with the heel first, but not on several of these factors simultaneously.

OBSTACLE CLEARANCE

For patients who tend to drag the foot on the affected side on the floor during swing phase, low and narrow obstacles are placed across the walking path at regular intervals corresponding to the patient's comfortable stride. Clearing such obstacles is not excessively difficult for patients with hemiplegia because the total flexor synergy may be utilized. But good judgment with respect to placement of the affected foot before lifting it over the obstacle is necessary, or the obstacle will be knocked down. A slow walking rhythm is maintained as the right and the left foot step over obstacles of equal height. For reasons of safety and to remove the patient's fear of falling, the physical therapist walks next to the patient, supporting him as described. The walking rhythm is maintained at the end of the obstacle course as both physical therapist and patient continue to step over imaginary obstacles that are described as becoming lower and lower until they are less than an inch high.

Clearing obstacles in walking is also recommended for patients with other types of gait deviations, and all patients should be given the opportunity to walk on and off carpets.

STAIRS

Methods of teaching stair walking need not be discussed in detail here, since physical therapists are usually familiar with this phase of the therapeutic program. The extent to which patients with hemiplegia may learn to manage stairs depends on the severity of the involvement and also on the availability of bannisters on one or both sides. For the student, it is well to remember that when stair walking is first attempted the patient's unaffected foot leads in ascending, the affected foot in descending; and that if a bannister is available only on the unaffected side when the patient ascends, he may have to descend backward.

MUSIC TO PROMOTE RHYTHM

A suitable melody played or hummed at the proper speed often aids the patient with hemiplegia to gain rhythm in walking; it is particularly enjoyed by patients in advanced recovery stages. Music may also prove useful for more fancy footwork, such as stepping forward, backward, and sideward, as in the practice of certain fundamental dance steps, all for the purpose of gaining better control of the affected limb. However, a fast rhythm may cause interference by spasticity and must be avoided. The response to music differs considerably among patients, hence its use should be selected accordingly.

REFERENCES

BEEVOR, C. E. Remarks on paralysis of movement of the trunk in hemiplegia. *Brit. Med. J.* 1909, i, p. 881. Edited and reprinted for the Guarantors of *Brain.* New York, Macmillan, 1951, p. 68.

BIRCH, H. G., PROCTOR, F., BORTNER, M., and LOWENTHAL, M. Perception in Hemiplegia: I. Judgment of vertical and horizontal by hemiplegic patients. *Arch. Phys. Med. 41:*19, 1960.

BIRCH, H. G., PROCTOR, F., BORTNER, M., and LOWENTHAL, M. Perception in hemiplegia: II. Judgment of the median plane. *Arch. Phys. Med. 41:*71, 1960.

BIRCH, H. G., PROCTOR, F., and BORTNER, M. Perception in hemiplegia: III. The judgment of relative distance in the visual field. *Arch. Phys. Med. 42:*639, 1961.

BRUELL, H. J., PESZCZYNSKI, M., and ALBEE, G. W. Disturbance of perception of verticality in patients with hemiplegia: A preliminary report. *Arch. Phys. Med.* 37:678, 1956.

BRUELL, H. J., PESZCZYNSKI, M., and VOLK, D. Disturbance of perception of verticality in patients with hemiplegia: Second report. *Arch. Phys. Med.* 38:776, 1957.

JACKSON, J. H. "Evolution and Dissolution of the Nervous System" (1884), in *Selected Writings of John Hughlings Jackson* ed. by J. Taylor. New York, Basic Books, 1958, p. 46.

SHERRINGTON, C. S. *The Integrative Action of the Nervous System,* 2nd ed. New Haven, Yale Univ. Press, 1947, p. 209.

Abstract 1

J. F. Bosma and E. Gellhorn

Electromyographic Studies of Muscular Coordination on Stimulation of the Motor Cortex

J. Neurophysiol. **9**:261–272, 1946

This study was undertaken to determine if co-contraction of antagonistic muscle pairs occurs under normal conditions, or if such co-contraction should be considered a pathological sign. The influence of variations of intensity and duration of stimuli is investigated.

METHODS AND MATERIAL

The experiments were conducted on normal, anesthetized animals (32 cats and 3 monkeys). The motor cortex of one of the cerebral hemispheres was exposed and stimulated with condenser discharges. The resulting action potentials were led off from flexor and extensor muscles by means of copper wires and, after amplification, were recorded with an Offner Inkwriter.

RESULTS

EFFECT OF INCREASE OF INTENSITY OF STIMULATION

A weak stimulation of the motor cortex had an *inhibitory* effect on flexor and/or extensor muscles, provided the electromyogram, prior to stimulation, showed a slight activity in the muscles.

A slight increase in intensity of stimulation resulted in increased activity of the stimulated muscle; simultaneously, its antagonist was inhibited. In other words, *reciprocal innervation* prevailed.

When the intensity of stimulation was further increased, the electromyogram showed activity of both flexor and extensor muscles; that is, *co-contraction* of agonistic and antagonistic muscles was present.

EFFECT OF INCREASE IN DURATION OF STIMULATION

At the onset of stimulation, *reciprocal innervation* was obtained; then, with prolonged stimulation, *co-contraction* of agonistic and antagonistic muscles developed.

The authors conclude:

"Indications are that with increasing number of discharging neurons the peripheral effect on individual muscles changes from inhibition to excitation, and in the case of an antagonistic pair of muscles, from inhibition to reciprocal innervation and finally to co-contraction (co-innervation). Under conditions of facilitation, the predominant type of coordination of fore- and hindleg muscles in flexor and extensor movements of moderate intensity is that of co-innervation."

Abstract 2

J. F. Bosma and E. Gellhorn

The Organization of the Motor Cortex of the Monkey, Based on Electromyographic Studies

Brain 70:127–144, 1947

This is a report on one in a series of studies on motor responses from cortical stimulation in monkeys, carried out at the Department of Physiology, University of Minnesota.

The present report concerns mainly the effects of prolonged stimulation of area 4 of the motor cortex with condenser discharges of slightly above-threshold intensities, as compared to brief supra-threshold stimuli.

Electromyographic records of activity in limb muscles were obtained by means of fine wire electrodes previously implanted in the following muscle pairs: biceps and triceps brachii; hamstrings and quadriceps femoris; flexor and extensor carpi radialis; and flexor and extensor carpi ulnaris. Multiple leads permitted the study of various combinations of muscular responses in the limbs.

The results obtained from the present as well as from a previous investigation (Murphy and Gellhorn, 1945) prompted the authors to repudiate the so-called "mosaic" or "punctuate" hypothesis of earlier investigators. According to this hypothesis, the motor cortex consists of a multitude of individual "tiles" which together form a mosaic, each "tile" representing an individual muscle. This hypothesis had been formulated because it had been found that very brief stimuli at specific points caused individual muscles to contract.

The studies reported here show that when stimulation time is prolonged (usually to 10 seconds) several muscles respond in specific combinations, or so-called "functional units." The authors postulate that cortical foci consist of bands in which neurons activating one muscle (such as the biceps brachii) are mixed with neurons activating other muscles (such as the extensor carpi muscles). The anatomical basis for neuromuscular coordination is believed to lie, to a large extent, in the intracortical connections existing between neurons which, although supplying different muscles, are located in the same cortical area. It is further postulated that functional units combine in numerous ways to form more complex movements, and that this applies to voluntary movement as well as to movements evoked by cortical stimulation.

Among functional units observed the following are mentioned:

1. The "biceps complex," a combination of the biceps brachii muscle and the extensor carpi muscles
2. The "triceps complex," a combination of the triceps muscles and the flexor carpi muscles
3. A combination of the hamstring muscles and the triceps complex

Well-defined patterns of movement were also evoked by stimulation of the motor cortex, namely:

1. *A progression pattern,* consisting of flexion of hip and knee and dorsiflexion of the ankle, in conjunction with retraction of the shoulder, extension of the elbow, and flexion of the wrist. (This combination is obtained in quadruped locomotion when the forelimb is in stance phase.)
2. *A grasping pattern,* characterized by protraction of the shoulder, flexion of the elbow, and closure of the fist.

The cortical locations for the zones which yielded the various functional units and patterns were mapped out in detail.

For instance, a medial zone of area 4 yielded response of the hamstring-triceps brachii complex. More laterally, the triceps combined with the flexor carpi muscle. The biceps complex was evoked from a medial zone of area 4. Between the foci for the triceps and the biceps complexes an area was found that yielded a biphasic response, that is, either the biceps complex developed first, followed by the triceps complex, or the response was in the opposite order.

When a specific functional unit is evoked, the antagonistic unit tends to become inhibited, but co-contraction of antagonistic muscles was also observed. When the biceps complex is evoked, co-contraction of the triceps is commonly seen. Upon activation of the triceps complex, however, co-contraction of the biceps brachii seldom occurs. This finding is interpreted as related to the great need for stabilization of elbow and wrist during grasping activities.

The authors stress that extensive additional electromyographic studies would be required for a more complete knowledge of the organization of the motor cortex, and that even if such knowledge were acquired "an important gap in our knowledge would still exist, since the modification of cortically induced movements by proprioceptive and other afferent impulses was not taken into account."

Remarks by S. Brunnstrom: This is one of the studies that furnishes the rationale for the facilitation techniques initiated by Dr. Herman Kabat and developed by Margaret Knott. Gellhorn's subsequent studies on the role of proprioception added several other principles to the techniques.

REFERENCES

Kabat, H. Studies on neuromuscular dysfunction: XV. The role of central facilitation in restoration of motor function in paralysis. *Arch. Phys. Med.* 33:521, 1952.

Knott, M., and Voss, D. E. *Proprioceptive Neuromuscular Facilitation. Patterns and Techniques.* 2nd ed. New York, Hoeber, 1968.

Murphy, J. P., and Gellhorn, E. Multiplicity of representation versus punctuate localization in the motor cortex. *Arch. Neurol. Psychiat.* 54:256, 1945.

Abstract 3

D. Denny-Brown

Disintegration of Motor Function Resulting from Cerebral Lesion

J. Nerv. Ment. Dis. *112*:1–45, 1950

The author delivered a highly interesting and informative Hughlings Jackson Lecture in Montreal in 1948, in which he stressed, among other things, that lesions of the Rolandic motor cortex do not produce paralysis of specific muscles, even if the lesion is very small, but rather a regional weakness; that topographical representation of muscles is relative, not absolute; that no one region of the central nervous system is alone responsible for motor synthesis of a specific motor act; and that a remarkable degree of restoration of motor function may occur in monkeys after ablation of areas 4 and 6 of the motor cortex.

The Rolandic motor cortex is of extreme importance for willed movement, but it is not the only cortical region concerned with motor acts. The importance of the extrarolandic cortex, of sensory cortical regions, and of the cerebellum is stressed: Neurological disorders of any one of these areas result in motor deficiency, hence it is evident that they all contribute to normal motor function.

Reference is made to Lashley's experiments on monkeys trained in motor skills. Skills acquired by these animals prior to lesions of area 4 of the motor cortex were so rapidly recovered that it was concluded that "electro-stimulable areas are rather more concerned with the maintenance of excitability and the regulation of postural reflexes than with the excitation and control of finely integrated movements" (Lashley 1924).

These observations by Lashley were substantiated by Denny-Brown's laboratory experiments. Following one-sided ablation of the Rolandic area in monkeys, considerable motor function recovered on the contralateral side.

To a large extent, the animal's motivation determined whether or not he would use the affected limb. Soon after ablation of the hand area, the affected hand was not used for grasping food, but when the animal was in fear of falling he would grasp weakly, and during angry spells his grasp became powerful. As recovery progressed, not only mass grasp but individual finger movements were performed, provided the motivation was strong. This was true of those animals whose entire contralateral hand and arm area had been ablated.

After partial recovery had taken place, additional cortical areas were ablated in stages until areas 4 and 6 had been destroyed on both sides. Severe depression of movement resulted, but the previously recovered movements were not abolished. Motor recovery was more rapid in proximal joints; but in the presence of a strong emotional stimulus, distal joint movement also returned.

Isolation of very small areas of the motor cortex for electrical stimulation revealed that these areas yielded responses of movement complexes, not of individual muscles. From a certain area, an extensive pattern response was evoked, involving upper and lower limbs on both sides. This pattern was also elicited from more caudal portions of the central nervous system. It is regarded as a basic motor pattern, a *bias,* or *anlage,* from which other motor responses have evolved.

The author presents evidence in support of the view that movement return following destruction of certain motor areas depends upon mechanisms that have been present all along as components of normal motor function; that is, there are no reasons to believe that an entirely new area has been activated to compensate for the destroyed area.

Further studies revealed that more motor recovery ensued after ablation of cortical motor areas than following pyramidal section. This indicates that extrapyramidal fibers contribute materially to the movement potential.

Evidence obtained from laboratory studies and clinical observations prompted the author to express the view that the Rolandic cortex "is concerned especially with the conditioning of proprioceptive stretch reflexes by contactual effects. The tactile components of this mechanism . . . has tonic, continued effects as well as special phasic and specific reactions. In the absence of this balance of tactile components in movement, the proprioceptive component is overactive, and this constitutes spasticity."

Neurological disorders, such as athetosis, dystonia, and tremor in Parkinson's disease, like the appearance of spasticity and rigidity, are each explained as a "disequilibrium due to loss of one member of a balanced pair."

REFERENCE

Lashley, K. S. Studies in cerebral function in learning 5. The retention of motor habits after destruction of the so-called motor areas in primates. *Arch. Neurol. Psychiat.* 12:249, 1924.

Abstract 4

E. Gellhorn

Patterns of Muscular Activity in Man

Arch. Phys. Med. 28:568–574, 1947

The number of muscles recruited for any one movement depends upon the effort exerted by the individual. With little effort, only the agonist is called into action; with more effort, antagonistic muscles also contract; and with increasing effort more and more muscles are activated. The present study was undertaken to investigate the relationship between the activities of wrist and elbow muscles.

METHODS

Twelve normal adult individuals, ages 20 to 30, participated. The subjects were seated with the arms supported in a horizontal position and the forearms stabilized. The elbow angle was kept at about 130 degrees, and the forearm was either pronated or supinated. Isometric contractions of the wrist flexor or the wrist extensor muscles were performed against resistance by springs of varying strength. The activities of the biceps brachii, the triceps brachii, the flexor carpi radialis, and the extensor carpi radialis muscles were recorded electromyographically by means of surface electrodes.

RESULTS

The electromyograms indicate that forceful isometric contractions of the wrist muscles (as agonists) evoke activity in the elbow muscles (as associated muscles). The patterns that evolve depend to a great extent on the position of the forearm, whether pronated or supinated.

Thus, the triceps brachii muscles become associated with the flexor carpi radialis muscle when the forearm is pronated, but with the extensor carpi radialis when the forearm is supinated.

The biceps brachii muscles become associated with the flexor carpi radialis muscle when the forearm is supinated, but with the extensor carpi radialis muscle when the forearm is pronated.

The functional significance of these four patterns become evident if the positions described and the direction of muscle action in each position are taken into consideration.

The action potentials that appeared in an associated muscle were, as a rule, of less amplitude than those of the agonist; in some instances, however, they equaled or even surpassed those of the agonist. The extent to which additional muscles were recruited, and co-contraction of antagonistic muscles appeared, varied considerably in individuals and depended upon the degree of effort exerted.

The author suggests that the above findings may be used to advantage for movement therapy, inasmuch as muscles that do not readily respond as agonists may become activated automatically as associated muscles.

Abstract 5

E. Gellhorn

The Influence of Alterations in Posture of the Limbs on Cortically Induced Movements

Brain 71:26–33, 1948

The purpose of this study on anesthetized monkeys was to determine in what manner, if any, changes in joint angles of a limb affect the motor responses resulting from stimulation of the motor cortex.

For example, before stimulation was applied the elbow was positioned either at an obtuse angle (biceps brachii lengthened, triceps brachii shortened) or at an acute angle (biceps brachii shortened, triceps brachii lengthened). A low-intensity current from condenser discharges was used, the ensuing movements were observed, and the activities of elbow and wrist muscles were recorded by electromyography. The same procedure was employed for the lower limb, where the position of the knee joint, or the ankle joint, was varied, and the activities of the muscles which control these joints were recorded.

RESULTS

UPPER LIMB

When a cortical flexor point was stimulated while the elbow joint was positioned at 120 degrees (obtuse angle), action potentials appeared in muscles of the "biceps complex," that is, in the biceps brachii and the extensor carpi muscles; rather surprisingly, the activity of the extensor carpi muscle was more intense than that of the biceps brachii. When the elbow was positioned at 45 degrees (acute angle) and the same flexor point was stimulated with the same intensity current, there was no response in the muscles of the biceps complex. Upon increase in duration of the stimulus, the extensor carpi muscle showed

minor activity of brief duration, but the biceps brachii still did not respond.

Stimulation of a cortical extensor point with the elbow at 65 degrees (triceps elongated) evoked responses in the muscles of the "triceps complex," that is, in the triceps brachii and the flexor carpi muscles. When the identical stimulus was applied at an elbow angle of 140 degrees, there was no response of the triceps brachii, but action potentials appeared in the flexor carpi muscle. If the same cortical point was stimulated with a higher intensity current, action potentials appeared also in the triceps brachii.

Wrist flexor and wrist extensor muscles could also be facilitated or inhibited by changing the wrist angle.

LOWER LIMB

Changes in joint angles of the lower limb had much the same effects as in the upper limb. With a knee angle of 160 degrees, the contraction of the hamstring muscles was facilitated, and that of the quadriceps muscles inhibited. When the knee joint was positioned at an acute angle and the identical stimulus was employed, the responses of the two muscle groups were reversed. Similar results were obtained from the tibialis anterior and the gastrocnemius muscles when the ankle was placed in dorsiflexion or plantar flexion.

In all the above experiments, the limb was positioned a few seconds before the stimulus was applied. Placing the limb in position as long as 5 minutes prior to cortical stimulation did not change the results; that is, no effect of temporal adaptation could be demonstrated.

CONCLUSIONS

When a muscle is elongated (all other factors being equal), its responsiveness to cortical stimulation increases in direct proportion to its length. The facilitating effect of muscular elongation on the activity of the muscle is explained as the result of an interaction between cortical impulses and proprioceptive impulses which originate in the elongated muscles. Whether this interaction takes place on the spinal or cortical level, or on both levels, was not determined.

The shunting of efferent impulses into pathways leading to elongated muscles as a result of proprioceptive messages arriving in the central nervous system was first observed by von Uexküll on nonvertebrates (see Abstract 25), then on decerebrate cats and dogs by Magnus (see Abstracts 12 and 13). This mechanism came to be known as the von Uexküll–Magnus rule. Gellhorn's studies demonstrate that this rule also applies to monkeys with intact nervous systems when motor responses are evoked from stimulation of the motor cortex.

Abstract 6

E. Gellhorn

Proprioception and the Motor Cortex

Brain 72:35–62, 1949

This study may be considered a continuation of earlier investigations dealing with the influence of proprioceptive impulses on the motor outcome resulting from cortical stimulation in monkeys. The present study is mainly concerned with the effects of fixation of one or more joints of a limb at various angles, so that muscles acting on these joints develop tension isometrically when they contract as a result of stimulation of the motor cortex.

The methods employed are similar to those described in earlier reports (see Bosma and Gellhorn, Abstract 2, and Gellhorn, Abstract 5). Low-intensity currents—at or slightly above threshold—are used, stimulation time is prolonged to 5 seconds or more, and the action potentials arising in the muscles are recorded electromyographically.

The article is profusely illustrated with electromyographic records that speak for themselves.

RESULTS

Figure 1 in the original article shows electromyograms of the inner hamstring muscles when the knee is fixated at 110 degrees, and of the same muscles at the same knee angle without fixation. In both instances, the identical stimulus is used at the identical cortical point. The amplitude of the electromyogram is considerably increased when the joint is fixated, as compared to that arising from the muscles when the joint is free to move.

In previous studies, elongation of a muscle had been shown to enhance its contraction. In the present study, therefore, it was desirable to consider the effect of elongation of a muscle as well as of fixation of the joint, and to determine which of these two factors predominates.

Figure 6 in the original article is a striking example of the combined effect of elongation of a muscle and fixation of the joint. In this experiment the ankle joint was fixated either in maximal plantar flexion or maximal dorsiflexion. The electromyograms from the tibialis anterior muscle show a remarkable increase in the amplitude when the ankle is in the plantar-flexed position. The electromyograms also show strong action potentials for several seconds following the cessation of the stimulus; that is, the after-discharge is marked.

The results of these and other experiments made it clear that proprioceptive impulses enhance the responsiveness to cortical stimulation, whether these impulses arise on account of joint fixation or muscle elongation. Of the two factors, joint fixation proved to be relatively more effective than muscle elongation.

The next step was to investigate the effect of proprioceptive impulses arising in a muscle, not only on the motor activity of that muscle, but also on the reactivity to cortical stimulation of muscles which form functional units with the first muscle. (See Bosma and Gellhorn, Abstract 2.)

For instance, a cortical flexor point was stimulated with the elbow fixated at 150 degrees and 30 degrees. At the former angle (biceps brachii elongated), the electromyogram of the biceps is of high amplitude, and so is that of the extensor carpi radialis muscle. At the acute angle, unfavorable for the biceps, the amplitudes of the electromyograms of the two muscles decrease (see Figure 13 of the original article). Thus, the two components of the biceps complex are influenced in the same direction.

The relationship of the components of the triceps complex was studied by stimulating a cortical extensor point. Proprioceptive impulses arising in the triceps brachii enhanced not only the muscular responses of this muscle, but also that of the flexor carpi radialis muscle. In addition, when the elbow angle was favorable for the triceps (45 degrees), the electromyograms showed that reciprocal innervation prevailed between antagonistic complexes, that is, increased activity of the triceps was accompanied by inhibition of the components of the biceps complex (see Figure 14 of the original article).

Although reciprocal innervation of antagonistic muscles was frequently observed in the above studies, co-contraction also occurred. In an earlier study (see Bosma and Gellhorn, Abstract 1), increase in intensity of a cortical stimulus had been shown to induce co-contraction (co-innervation) of antagonistic muscles. It was now demonstrated that such co-contraction also results from interaction of a weak cortical stimulus with strong proprioceptive impulses.

Important results of the present studies are summarized, in part, as follows:

"Fixation of a muscle at increased length greatly increases the response of this muscle if the proper cortical focus is chosen. This effect is largely due to impulses set up while the muscle develops tension isometrically.

"Proprioceptive impulses thus induced become effective, although to a lesser extent, in those muscles with which the proprioceptively excited muscle forms specific functional associations.

"These effects seem to be based on the interaction of proprioceptive impulses with those elicited by cortical stimulation, resulting in an increased number of discharging motor units."

The author suggests that proprioceptive-cortical facilitation as demonstrated in this study be employed in movement therapy for patients with central lesions.

Abstract 7

K. E. Hagbarth

Excitatory and Inhibitory Skin Areas for Flexor and Extensor Motoneurones

Acta Physiol. Scand. **26**, Suppl. 94, Stockholm, 1952, 58 pp.

Sherrington's flexion reflex is readily evoked by cutaneous stimuli applied to the fore- or hindlimb of an animal. The receptive field for the flexion reflex of the hindlimb includes the skin of the entire limb, from the toes distally to the groin proximally. The lowest threshold of excitation is found in distal areas (see Sherrington, Abstract 20).

Although flexion responses are the rule, certain ipsilateral extension responses may also be observed. For example, Sherrington describes an *extensor thrust* that is elicited by pressure on the toe-pads of a spinal dog. More recent studies indicate that other types of ipsilateral extension reflexes may be evoked within the receptive field of the flexion reflex.

In the present publication, Hagbarth reports on a systematic investigation of the distribution of skin receptors facilitating and inhibiting flexor and extensor motoneurones in the hindlimb of the cat.

A number of different approaches were utilized. In many of the experiments the effects of cutaneous "conditioning" stimuli on monosynaptic spinal cord reflexes (in terms of facilitation or inhibition) were explored. The experimental animals were decerebrated, and in many cases the spinal cord was sectioned in the lower thoracic region. The anterior spinal roots of L5 to S2 on one side were dissected free and severed; the central stumps were used for recording efferent impulses, the reflex being evoked from a muscle nerve on the ipsilateral side. The muscle nerve was usually isolated (severed), but in some instances were left intact. The conditioning stimuli were applied either directly to the skin or to a cutaneous nerve prepared for such

purpose. Usually, the contralateral limb was denervated. Antagonistic muscle pairs were chosen for the investigation, namely: *at ankle*, calf muscles and tibialis anterior; *at knee*, semitendinosus and quadriceps femoris (rectus removed); *at toes*, extensor brevis digitorum and flexor brevis digitorum.

When the conditioning shock was applied to a nerve trunk, varying efferent effects were obtained which led the author to conclude that "In the cutaneous nerve trunks afferent fibers from different skin areas are intermingled and therefore sensory components with opposite reflex function are indiscriminately activated by stimuli to such nerves." The reflex response represents "some state of balance of opposite influences."

The effects of conditioning stimuli applied directly to the skin proved much easier to interpret. For this investigation the cutaneous nerve trunks were left intact and the skin was stimulated by a pinch between the thumb and the fingers, or a small forceps was used. The test reflexes were evoked from the nerves to the extensor muscles. By methodically pinching the skin in all regions of the limb, the areas of excitation and inhibition for each of the extensor muscles were mapped out.

The results in terms of excitation and inhibition of motoneurones of flexor and extensor muscles at ankle and knee were as follows:

Tibialis anterior muscle: Inhibited from the skin over the heel and posterior leg, excited from all other areas.

Calf muscles: Excited from the skin over the heel and posterior leg, inhibited from all other areas.

Semitendinosus muscle: Inhibited from the

skin just below the knee, over the knee, and over the entire anterior thigh, excited from all other areas.

Quadriceps femoris muscles (vasti): Excited from the skin just below the knee, over the knee, and over the entire anterior thigh, inhibited from all other areas.

The field for excitation of flexor muscles was thus quite extensive, as already noticed by Sherrington (see Abstract 20). *The field for excitation of extensor motoneurones was limited to the skin overlying the extensor muscles and their tendinous insertions.* The excitation produced in one extensor muscle did not spread to other extensor muscles; the effect was strictly *local*.

Because the stimulus employed (pinching of the skin) is adequate for many different skin receptors, the author endeavored to find out which of the end-organs were mainly responsible for the effects observed.

Moderate pressure to a shaven skin area, or light touch to an unshaven area over the calf muscles, if effective at all, was always excitatory for the calf muscles. Moderate changes in temperature to the same area did not evoke any observable reflex effects, but excessive heat had an excitatory effect. The conclusion was reached that nociceptive nerve endings and, to a certain extent, tactile end-organs are involved, but that nerve endings responding to changes in temperature are of less importance.

CONCEALED EFFECTS

Although each skin area yielded either excitation or inhibition of flexor or extensor motoneurones, it was demonstrated that effects of opposite character may be present in the same area. Because of the dominance of one type of effects, however, the opposite effect becomes concealed.

Abstract 8

K. E. Hagbarth

Spinal Withdrawal Reflexes in Human Lower Limb

J. Neurol., Neurosurg. Psychiat. 23:222-227, 1960

In a previous study (Hagbarth, Abstract 7), excitatory and inhibitory skin areas for flexor and extensor motoneurones in the lower limb of the cat were mapped out, and the results compared to the receptive field for the flexion reflex, as described by Sherrington (Abstract 20).

The present study was undertaken to determine the effects of stimulation of the skin in various areas of the lower human limb in terms of excitation and inhibition of flexor and extensor motoneurones.

The subjects were normal adult males. Brief electrical stimuli causing an intense burning sensation and resulting in a withdrawal response were applied to the skin. The muscular responses were recorded electromyographically by means of bipolar needle electrodes. By having the subjects maintain a slight voluntary tension in the muscles examined, inhibitory as well as excitatory effects could be assessed from the electromyograms.

The preliminary experiments of this study concerned the effect of noxious stimuli applied to the most distal part of the limb (plantar surface of hallux), which area in Sherrington's animal experiments proved to have the lowest threshold of excitation for the flexion reflex.

The results, as revealed by the electromyograms, indicated excitation of the following muscles: tensor fasciae femoris,* sartorius, rectus femoris, tibialis anterior, peroneus longus, extensor digitorum brevis. Inhibition was recorded in gluteus maximus, vastus medialis, vastus lateralis, gastrocnemius, soleus and flexor digitorum brevis. The semimembra-

nosus muscle was usually associated with the extensor muscles, the semitendinosus with the flexor muscles, but the responses of these two muscles varied somewhat.

The flexion reflex was followed by "silent periods" of the flexor muscles. The extensor muscles often exhibited secondary discharges and sometimes recurrent inhibitions and excitations.

The latencies of the responses were very short (60 to 80 msec.), which led to the conclusion that in man as in animals the flexion response is a true spinal cord reflex. Furthermore, the author points out, the muscles activated in the flexion reflex in man are practically identical with those participating in the flexion reflex in animals (Sherrington, Abstract 20).

The main study consisted of a systematic investigation of the effects of noxious stimuli applied to the anterior and posterior surfaces of the entire limb on the excitability status of the extensor muscles (gluteus maximus, vastus medialis, and calf muscles). The results were as follows:

Gluteus maximus muscle: "Inhibited from most skin areas but it regularly responded with a brisk initial reflex discharge to skin stimuli in the gluteal region."

Vastus medialis muscle: "Inhibited from most skin areas of the limb, including the gluteal region, but usually initial discharges appeared when the ventral part of the thigh was stimulated."

Gastrocnemius and soleus muscles: "Excited from skin area of the posterior side of the limb, from the heel to just above the knee." Inhibition was obtained from the skin over the foot and the anterior surface of the leg. No effect was obtained from the skin over the quadriceps and over the gluteus maximus muscles.

* *Remarks by S. Brunnstrom:* Hagbarth uses (as Sherrington did) the older term, "tensor fasciae femoris," instead of the newer nomenclature, "tensor fasciae latae."

SUMMARY

"Besides the patterns of the flexion reflex there are local extension reflexes which are mainly elicitable from skin areas covering extensor muscles. It is believed that these local extension reflexes serve a protective purpose in that they can cause an effective withdrawal of the heel, knee and buttock, especially when the limb supports the body weight."

F. A. Hellebrandt, S. J. Houtz, D. E. Hockman, and M. J. Partridge

Physiological Effects of Simultaneous Static and Dynamic Exercise

Amer. J. Phys. Med. 35:106–117, 1956

In previous years, the main author and her associates studied the work capacity of the wrist extensor muscles when they were exercised against heavy resistance until extremely fatigued, either unilaterally, alternately left and right, reciprocally, or synchronously (Hellebrandt and associates, 1950, 1951). The subjects—well-trained and well-motivated young men and women—were seated with the pronated forearms supported on a table and the hands protruding over the edge of the table. The work output was measured by means of an ergograph as the load was repeatedly raised a prescribed distance at a cadence set by a metronome, usually in bouts of 25. When the muscles became fatigued, the load could no longer be raised the entire range at the prescribed cadence—that is, the work output declined. By multiplying the distance through which the load was raised by the weight of the load for each stroke and adding the results of the 25 strokes, the work output per bout was obtained.

These studies demonstrated that the work output on the exercising side was enhanced when the contralateral side was also exercised, and that this facilitating influence became marked during fatigue. In one type of experiment, the exercising side performed alone on odd bouts while the two sides performed synchronously on even bouts. During bilateral performance, a "revival" of power on the fatigued side was regularly observed.

The present investigation concerns the effect on work output of simultaneous static and dynamic exercise of the wrist extensor muscles. The experimental conditions were essentially the same as during the earlier studies. Both ergographic and electromyographic records were obtained.

During a single bout of heavily resisted wrist extension on one side, the subject's task was to maintain an ergographic load at a certain height on the contralateral side. When the load on the holding side was extremely heavy, it could only be held at full height momentarily; thereafter, in spite of the subject's maximal effort of resistance, it began to descend. A record of the descent was supplied by the ergograph. On the exercising side the work output was measured ergographically with a load sufficiently heavy to produce rapid exhaustion. When the records thus obtained were compared with the control records (obtained from unilateral performances) it became evident that the static effort was enhanced by simultaneous dynamic work. The authors state: "The mean height of the static contraction was higher and the load was sustained for a longer interval of time when dynamic work was being done concurrently. . . . The magnitude of the effect was on the order of 40 per cent. Dynamic work also increased but to a somewhat lesser degree. It was observed repeatedly that, when the non-preferred hand performed its normal holding function, it was less affected by dynamic activity of the dominant limb than the reverse procedure."

It is pointed out that facilitatory effects of simultaneous static and dynamic exercise is only obtained in well-trained individuals. Less well-coordinated persons may find it difficult, even confusing, to carry out different types of exercises on the two sides, in which case an inhibitory rather than a facilitatory effect may be expected.

In another experiment, when dynamic work was performed in repeated bouts with a moderately heavy load, the influence of static holding on the fatigue curve of the exercising side became well demonstrable. Odd bouts of dynamic work were performed without static holding; on even bouts the contralateral side assumed its holding function. In one experiment (graphically illustrated), the percentage decrement in work output on the fourteenth bout was approximately 20 per cent less than on the fifteenth bout, and approximately 30 per cent less than on the sixteenth bout.

The electromyograms show, first, that volitional wrist extension against heavy resistance is accompanied by strong contraction of the biceps brachii muscle, confirming a pattern described by Gellhorn (see Abstract 4). Second, that static holding is performed more steadily by the nondominant hand, while the dominant hand performs dynamic work, than when the procedure is reversed.

SUMMARY (IN PART)

1. "Simultaneous static and dynamic work is mutually facilitatory in the trained subject."
2. "The magnitude of the facilitatory effort is related to the severity of the effort."
3. "Action patterns evoked in the dominant cortex affect the contralateral holding hand less than those elicited by repetitive contraction of the non-preferred extremity."

REFERENCES

Hellebrandt, F. A., Houtz, S. J., and Krikorian, A. M. Influence of bimanual exercise on unilateral work capacity. *J. Appl. Physiol.* 2:446–452, 1950.

Hellebrandt, F. A., Houtz, S. J., and Eubank, R. N. Influence of alternate and reciprocal exercise on work capacity. *Arch. Phys. Med.* 32:766–776, 1951.

Abstract 10

F. A. Hellebrandt, S. J. Houtz, M. J. Partridge, and C. E. Walters

Tonic Neck Reflexes in Exercises of Stress in Man

Amer. J. Phys. Med. 35:144–159, 1956

The purpose of the study was to observe postural patterns resulting from stressful volitional movements in man, to investigate the biological significance of these patterns, and to assess their usefulness for therapeutic procedures.

MATERIAL AND METHODS

Eighteen highly motivated adult subjects (nine male, nine female) participated, four of whom were cerebral palsied individuals. The subjects were seated and performed repetitive wrist movements of flexion or extension against increasing resistance in bouts usually of 25 contractions. Rest periods between bouts equal in duration to the active phase were given. The exercise continued until the subjects were exhausted and could no longer perform in the prescribed manner.

A modification of the Mosso ergograph was used to trace the excursions of the movements; from the ergographic record the work output was calculated in gram centimeters. The activities of flexor and extensor muscles of wrist and elbow and of selected shoulder and neck muscles were recorded by electromyography by means of surface electrodes. Some experiments were performed unilaterally, others bilaterally. In both types of experiments the influence of the tonic neck reflex was studied.

ERGOGRAPHIC STUDIES

When the subjects voluntarily rotated the head toward and away from the exercising side on alternate bouts, the ergograms clearly indicated an effect of the head position on work output in the normal subjects. The effect was much more marked in the cerebral palsied subjects.

For example, the work output in gram centimeters during *wrist extension* (the weaker of the two wrist movements) in four consecutive bouts in a normal and in a cerebral palsied subject was as follows:

	1[*]	2[†]
Normal subject	1,276	1,395
	1,188	1,318
	2,464	2,712
Cerebral palsied subject	81	224
	87	203
	168	427

Facilitatory and inhibitory effects of head positioning on work output during *wrist flexion* was also present but it was less marked than on wrist extension (example for normal subject not given):

	1[*]	2[†]
Cerebral palsied subject	884	828
	1,132	684
	2,016	1,512

In other similar experiments, heavily resisted flexion or extension wrist movements were performed bilaterally, with the head either ventroflexed or dorsiflexed.

During *bilateral wrist flexion*, ventroflexion

---

[*] Head rotated away from the exercising side.
[†] Head rotated toward the exercising side.

of the head (and neck) augmented work output, while dorsiflexion had the opposite effect. During *bilateral wrist extension,* dorsiflexion of the head augmented work output, and ventroflexion had the opposite effect. All effects increased with progressively increasing fatigue.

It was thus demonstrated that the rules governing the tonic neck reflexes, as formulated by Magnus and de Kleijn for decerebrate animals (see Abstract 16), are applicable also to human subjects.

ELECTROMYOGRAPHIC STUDIES

During the ergographic studies records of the activities of a number of antagonistic muscle groups of both upper limbs were obtained by electromyography. Multiple leads from surface electrodes were used. The following outlines some of the findings.

STAGES OF MUSCULAR INVOLVEMENT

1. During the first portion of unilateral wrist exercise, no evidence of muscular activity on the contralateral side was detected. On the exercising side, the agonist was quite active and its antagonist slightly active.

2. With increasing stress, first the contralateral antagonist, then the contralateral agonist, became active.

3. Toward the end of the exercise, shortly before exhaustion, electrical activity on both sides of the body became marked, in agonists as well as antagonists. Muscles sampled bilaterally, in addition to the wrist muscles, were flexor and extensor muscles of elbow, anterior and posterior deltoid muscles, sternocleidomastoid muscles, and upper trapezius muscles. The authors state that during this last stage of exercise "it is difficult to detect, from the electromyogram alone, which of the muscles sampled are performing voluntarily and which participate reflexly. This is the so-called agony phase of an all-out effort. It is attained only

by well-trained subjects, thoroughly inured to the discomfort of severe exercise."

PATTERNS OF MUSCULAR PARTICIPATION

It was demonstrated that the tone of the neck muscles, especially that of the sternocleidomastoid muscle, was influenced by wrist exercise. As an example, wrist flexion on the right side (without asymmetrical head positioning) resulted in action potentials in the right sternocleidomastoid muscle. When the wrist flexion exercise changed to the left side, electrical activity of the left sternocleidomastoid muscle appeared. *An influence from limb to neck* was thus demonstrated, while experiments with voluntary head positioning had shown an influence *from neck to limb.*

As stress increased, it was observed that the head moved spontaneously into a position which facilitated the task. Thus afferent impulses originating in the exercising limb caused the head to be positioned, the head position evoked the tonic neck reflex, and the reflex enhanced the muscular performance.

In the original article line drawings of typical symmetrical and asymmetrical body attitudes assumed spontaneously during forceful wrist exercise are reproduced, with corresponding electromyograms. It is demonstrated that increased effort in the performance of wrist movements causes muscular activity to spread, not only to the contralateral upper limb and to the neck, but also to abdomen, back, and even to muscles of the lower limbs.

CONCLUSIONS

"We conclude . . . that reflexes arising in the limbs themselves during heavy resistance exercise in man regulate the posture of the head, and this in turn expedites performance, adding another to the gamut of indirect or reflex training techniques now being used in the clinic for the rehabilitation of the disabled."

John Hughlings Jackson

Selected Writings of John Hughlings Jackson

J. Taylor, ed., New York, Basic Books, 1958

John Hughlings Jackson is perhaps best known for his investigations of epilepsy and its after-effects. A common type of epilepsy is named after him (Jacksonian epilepsy). Jackson was a keen clinical observer, a prominent scientist, a philosopher, and a prolific writer.[*]

Jackson postulates that through pathological processes the nervous system, or part of it, is reduced to an earlier developmental stage. This hypothesis is discussed in many of his writings and was the subject of his Croonian Lectures, entitled "Evolution and Dissolution of the Nervous System," delivered at the Royal College of Physicians in March, 1884.

Dissolution means a reversal of evolution. In Jackson's words, "Evolution is a passage from the most simple to the most complex, from the most automatic to the most voluntary. Dissolution is a process of undevelopment; it is a 'taking to pieces' in order, from the most complex and most voluntary, toward the most simple and most automatic." Since, in pathology of the nervous system, evolution is not completely reversed, some level of evolution remains. Therefore, "to undergo dissolution" may also be expressed as "to be reduced to a lower level of evolution" (p. 46).[†]

Basing his theories on the doctrine of evolution, Jackson outlines the hierarchy of the nervous system as consisting of *lowest, middle,* and *highest centers,* which represent the evolution from the most automatic to the most voluntary. These centers are not altogether synonymous with morphological divi-

[*] A list of his publications, which appeared over a period of 48 years (1861–1909), is found in *Selected Writings,* Vol. II.

[†] Page numbers given in this abstract refer to *Selected Writings,* Vol. II.

sions of the nervous system; they must be regarded as anatomicophysiological units.

Throughout the discussions, the intimate relations between sensory and motor centers are stressed. "The whole nervous system is a sensori-motor mechanism, a coordinating system from top to bottom" (p. 41).

The *lowest motor centers* are represented by the anterior horns of the spinal cord and the nuclei for the cranial nerves. Muscles in all parts of the body are here represented, but in few movement combinations only. The lowest centers are responsible for the simplest, most automatic, and least voluntary motor acts. With the corresponding sensory centers, they constitute the lowest level of the nervous system.

The *middle motor centers* are found in the Rolandic region. All the muscles represented on the lowest level are here rerepresented in a more complex manner, so that a great variety of muscle combinations that are less automatic and more voluntary become possible. With the corresponding sensory centers, the middle motor centers constitute the middle level of the nervous system.

The *highest motor centers* are believed to be located in the frontal lobe, anterior to the middle centers. With the corresponding sensory centers, they make up the third or highest level of the nervous system. The highest motor centers represent, in a still more complex manner, the body parts which the middle centers have represented. They are thus re-re-representing muscles of the entire body (p. 42). The highest level of the nervous system is said to constitute the anatomical basis for consciousness, the "organ of the mind."

Dissolution of the nervous system may involve the entire system or have a local character. Any one of the three levels may be affected locally.

The common type of hemiplegia, caused by a lesion in the middle motor centers, is given as an example of local dissolution. "There is loss of more or fewer of the most voluntary movements of one side of the body; we find that the arm, the more voluntary limb, suffers more and longer; we find, too, that the most voluntary part of the face suffers more than the rest of the face." A lower level of evolution, however, remains in hemiplegia. It may be observed that unilateral movements are largely lost, while bilateral movements which are more automatic may be retained.

Aphasia is cited as another example of local dissolution. "There is loss of the intellectual language with persistence of emotional, the more automatic language." For example, swearing, an emotional language, is often retained by hemiplegic patients. And, if you ask the aphasic, "Is your name Jones?", he may reply, "No." But if you ask him to say "no," he may be unable to do so, because then voluntary control is required (p. 49).

Aphasia is discussed extensively in a number of Jackson's publications, notably in an article entitled "On Affections of the Speech from Disease of the Brain," first published in 1878 (see p. 155).

There are positive and negative aspects of each type of dissolution. In hemiplegia, for example, there is loss of control of muscles, a negative symptom, because of the lesion in the internal capsule. Simultaneously, there is a tonic condition of the muscles, a positive symptom. "Negative states of the nervous centers cannot *cause* positive states of muscles, they may *permit* them" (p. 452). Spasticity in hemiplegia (Jackson's term is *rigidity*) is explained as the unantagonized influence of other nervous centers. Normality requires a state of balance between opposing forces, a conception which Jackson expresses as "cooperation of antagonists."

Remarks by S. Brunnstrom: The influence of Jackson's thinking is evident in much of the neurological literature to this day. Although neurophysiological research since Jackson's days may have disproved some of his speculations with respect to the details of the function of the nervous system, his main themes have proved to be of lasting value. Jackson was not only a keen clinical observer, but his writings reveal a remarkable insight into the intricate function of the nervous system and a vision which foretold discoveries to come. He was indeed a great man.

Abstract 12

R. Magnus

Zur Regelung der Bewegungen durch das Zentralnervensystem, I. Mitteilung (The Regulation of Movements by the Central Nervous System Part 1 [Experiments on spinal dogs])

Pflüger Arch. Physiol. 130:219–252, 1909

Experiments were undertaken on spinal dogs to determine whether or not von Uexküll's rule for nonvertebrates applies also to higher animals.

It was demonstrated that reflexes of the hindlimbs were markedly influenced by the initial positions of the joints of the responding limb. If the initial position of the limb was flexion, an extensor response was obtained. Conversely, if the initial position was extension, a flexor response ensued. Reversal of direction of a crossed reflex could thus be obtained by changing the initial position of the limb.

Three types of stimuli were used to elicit a crossed reflex, namely: (1) striking the patellar tendon; (2) striking the bone above or below the knee; and (3) administering a painful stimulus to the limb.

1. CROSSED REFLEXES ELICITED BY STRIKING THE PATELLAR TENDON

By briskly tapping the patellar tendon on the right side, extension of the right knee is obtained; simultaneously, an extensor reflex (extension of the knee, usually also of the hip) is elicited on the left side. This crossed response is obtained regularly, provided the left limb is flexed or semiflexed at the time the stimulus is applied. But if the left limb is extended prior to the application of the stimulus, the left limb flexes. In the original article,

frames of motion pictures illustrating these results are shown.

It is thus demonstrated that the identical stimulus may produce opposite results, depending upon the posture of the responding limb; that is, a reflex reversal (Reflexumkehr) may be induced. Since different results may be obtained from the identical stimulus, a *shunting* (Schaltung) of efferent impulses into this or that pathway apparently takes place in the spinal cord, effected by afferent impulses originating in the crossed limb.

The latency of the crossed extensor reflex averaged 0.09 second; of the crossed flexor reflex, 0.06 second (average of five determinations). The latency of the flexor response was thus found to be somewhat shorter than that of the extensor response.

The relative importance of the positions of hip, knee, and ankle joints in determining the pattern of the crossed reflex was investigated. In Table I in the original publication the results are given of 93 experiments, four different starting positions of the crossed limb being used, namely:

1. Hip flexed, knee and ankle extended.
2. Hip extended, knee and ankle flexed.
3. Hip and knee flexed, ankle extended.
4. Hip and ankle extended, knee flexed.

The results of these various combinations of joint positions were not always uniform, but as a rule those muscles which were most elongated responded. The hip joint was found to be by far the most influential in determining the outcome of the pattern of the entire limb.

2. BONE REFLEXES

If by mistake the bone above or below the knee joint is tapped instead of the patellar tendon, the reaction occurs in the same manner as if the tendon had been hit. It is pointed out that crossed extension of the knee resulting from striking the femoral condyle was already reported by Philippson. Magnus demonstrated that Philippson's reflex could be reversed in the manner described above.

3. CROSSED REFLEXES ELICITED BY PAINFUL STIMULI

A pinprick on one of the toe pads of the animal's hindlimb or some other painful stimulus to the limb elicits a withdrawal movement of the entire limb (Sherrington's nociceptive flexor reflex). Simultaneously, the contralateral limb extends. A firm functional relation exists between these two reflexes—flexion on one side, extension on the other side. In spite of the strong linkage of the two reflexes, Magnus was able to demonstrate that reversal of the crossed reflex could be obtained by changing the initial position of the crossed limb. It is of special interest to note that a functional linkage of such strength can be broken and changed into an opposite reaction, which indicates that the linkage between the two reflexes is not an absolute one.

(This report by Magnus also discusses other reflexes, such as the extensor thrust and the scratch reflex, as well as the influence of general anesthesia, shock, and illness on the various reflexes.)

The muscle elongation principle discovered by von Uexküll thus was found to be applicable also to mammals (see also Part 2, dealing with experiments on cats).

REFERENCE

Philippson, M. L'autonomie et la centralisation dans le système nerveux des animaux. *Trav. Lab. Inst. Physiol., Inst. Solvay* 7:1–208, 1905.

Abstract 13

R. Magnus

Zur Regelung der Bewegungen durch das Zentralnervensystem, II. Mitteilung (The Regulation of Movements by the Central Nervous System Part 2 [Tail reflexes in spinal cat])

Pflüger Arch. Physiol. 130:253–269, 1909

The tail of the cat is considered the "classical object" for demonstrating reflex reversal in higher animals. For the present investigation, spinal cats, first decerebrated, are employed.

The cat's tail is a jointed column, moveable in all directions. The tail vertebrae are connected by four groups of muscles which function as extensors (elevators), flexors (depressors), and side abductors. Muscles also connect the root of the tail with the pelvis, the sacrum, and the lumbar vertebrae.

Vivid tail reflexes may be elicited by stimulating various regions of the skin and by pressure on the vertebral column. The most convenient point to apply the stimulus is the tip of the tail. In some animals it suffices to touch the hair of the tip of the tail with one finger; in other animals a pinching of the tip of the tail is required to evoke a response.

If the experimental animal is held in a vertical position, head up, and the tail hangs straight down, stimulation of the tip of the tail results in irregularly directed reflex responses—that is, the tail movements may occur to the left or right, or in a dorsal or ventral direction. It is immaterial if the tail is pinched in a dorsoventral or side-to-side direction. Stimuli in the lumbar region, whether on the right or the left side, also elicit unpredictable responses, not necessarily toward the side that is stimulated.

As soon as the tail position is no longer symmetrical, the reflex movements follow a definite rule: they always occur toward the side of the elongated muscles. This rule was demonstrated by numerous experiments.

The cat may be positioned on its side (right or left) with the tail hanging over the edge of the table so that the root of the tail is markedly bent and the rest of the tail hangs almost vertically. In this position, stimulation of the tip of the tail always causes the tail to move in an upward direction by the abductor muscles on the right or on the left side. In the original article frames of motion pictures are reproduced which show that the tail movement begins at the root of the tail where the bend of the tail is most marked, then proceeds distally as other muscles gradually become elongated. The illustrations show the reactions of the animal placed on its left and on its right sides.

It was demonstrated that the elongation rule also applies to the muscles which move the tail in a dorsoventral direction. The cat was held with the head downward, and the tail was allowed to hang either toward the animal's abdomen or toward its back. In the first instance, a tail stimulus evoked a dorsally directed response, in the latter instance a ventrally directed response.

Tail reflexes were observed in 25 different experimental animals and during more than 300 individual experiments. The tail responses consistently took place toward the side of the elongated muscles.

The author points out that with respect to anatomical arrangements, the tail of the cat is

151

comparable to the arm of the starfish in von Uexküll's experiments (see Abstract 25). In the starfish, the direction of the reflex responses was found to depend upon two factors: the side on which the stimulus was applied and the state of the muscles with respect to elongation. Magnus demonstrated that in the case of the tail of the cat, the choice of site of stimulation had practically no influence on the outcome of the reflex, which was totally determined by the state of elongation of the tail muscles.

Magnus' experiments show that afferent impulses originating at the periphery and flowing into the spinal cord may be transmitted to many different motor centers, resulting in a variety of motor responses, as when the tail is in a symmetrical position with respect to the vertebral column. But when the tail deviates from the symmetrical position, the impulses are regularly shunted to those motor centers which correspond to the elongated muscles.

The author does not venture at this time to explain the exact mechanism of the above shunting. Is it the elongation of the muscles that causes the shunting, he asks, or are afferent impulses from joints and skin equally, or exclusively, responsible?*

---

* *Remarks by S. Brunnstrom:* Subsequent studies by Magnus supplied the answers to these questions. It was found that afferent impulses from joints and skin areas could be eliminated without affecting the motor outcome. But if afferent nerves from the elongated muscles were severed, the shunting phenomenon ceased. It was concluded that proprioceptive impulses from muscles, tendons, and fascia were responsible for shunting the efferent impulses into pathways leading to the elongated muscles. (See Magnus' book, *Körperstellung,* Berlin, Springer, 1924, Chap. II, p. 42.)

R. Magnus

Some Results of Studies in the Physiology of Posture Cameron Price Lectures Part I.

Lancet 211(2):531–536, 1926

PART I

Part I deals with (1) local static reactions —the positive supporting reaction and the negative supporting reaction; (2) segmental reactions, such as the crossed extension reflex and the "Schunkelreflex;" (3) general static reactions of the decerebrate preparation, such as the tonic neck and labyrinthine reflexes.

POSITIVE SUPPORTING REACTION

A normal animal is capable of using his limbs for a variety of nonweight-bearing activities, such as scraping, digging, scratching, and fighting, but at other times the limb is transferred to a "stiff pillar" for the purpose of supporting body weight. This transformation is brought about by a series of local reflexes which together constitute the positive supporting reaction. Both normal and "thalamus animals" exhibit this reaction.

When a dog is lying on its side, usually no resistance to passive flexion of the limb is felt. But if the limb is extended and the investigator dorsiflexes the animal's paw and exerts pressure against the toe pads, a strong extensor response is obtained—the limb no longer permits passive flexion. The muscular tension thus evoked suffices to maintain body weight when the animal is turned around to the standing position.

The afferent impulses which evoke the reflex originate in part from *proprioceptors* in the stretched muscles, in part from *exteroceptors* from contact with the toe pads. Experiments with decerebrate dogs in the supine position show that exteroceptors alone may suffice to evoke the reflex. A light touch of the

toe pads without dorsiflexion of the paw evoked a strong response. It appeared to the investigator "as though the slowly extending foot were being drawn after the receding finger by some magnetic force." (The phenomenon is referred to as the "magnet reaction.") Cutting the cutaneous nerves to the foot abolished the reaction.

It was demonstrated that during the positive supporting reaction *flexor and extensor muscles contracted simultaneously*. This is in contradistinction to other reflexes such as the crossed extension reflex, which is characterized by reciprocal innervation. Because of co-contraction of antagonistic pairs of muscles during the positive supporting reaction, the joints become firmly stabilized.

THE NEGATIVE SUPPORTING REACTION

This reaction affects the tension of the muscles of the limb in the opposite direction from that of the positive supporting reaction. When the limb is lifted off the ground the paw flexes, and this movement evokes relaxation of the previously tense muscles throughout the limb: the limb becomes free to move.

THE CROSSED EXTENSION REFLEX

In the symmetrical standing position the animal's body weight is carried by all four limbs. A painful stimulus to one of the limbs —for example, a hindlimb—evokes a withdrawal reflex of that limb and also extension of the hindlimb on the opposite side. The purpose of the crossed extension reflex is to reinforce the positive supporting reaction by increasing the tension in the extensor muscles of the limb which now has to carry additional weight.

THE SHIFTING REACTION

This reflex is similar in nature to the crossed extension reflex. It may be demonstrated in normal animals as well as in animals whose forebrain and cerebellum have been removed. It is also present in man.

When one of the limbs of an animal—for example, the right forelimb—is lifted off the ground during the negative supporting reaction and the investigator moves the animal's thorax toward the right, an increased tension in the extensor muscles of the right elbow is felt; then the entire limb becomes fully extended for the purpose of preventing a fall toward that side. The same reaction is also present in the hindlimb.

If a human subject is standing on one foot and the body weight is moved toward the unsupported side, the lifted leg is automatically lowered to the ground to prevent a fall. This reaction can hardly be inhibited by will.

The "Schunkelreflex" originates in the proprioceptors of the adductor muscles of the stance limb as these muscles are being elongated by the shifting of the body weight toward the unsupported side.

In animals, a similar "Schunkelreflex" is evoked if the animal's body is moved in a forward or backward direction.

Part I of this publication also discusses decerebrate rigidity, first described by Sherrington in 1898 (see Abstract 18), and the tonic neck and labyrinthine reflexes of Magnus and de Kleijn (see Abstract 15).

Abstract 15

R. Magnus

Some Results of Studies in the Physiology of Posture Cameron Price Lectures Part II.

Lancet 211(2):585–588, 1926

PART II: GENERAL STATIC REACTIONS OF THE MIDBRAIN ANIMAL

Decerebrate rigidity results from transection of the brainstem anywhere caudal to the midbrain but rostral to the entrance of the eighth nerves into the medulla. The results vary somewhat, depending upon the exact location of the cut. When the transection approaches the midbrain, the *neck-righting reflexes* appear while decerebrate rigidity persists. But when the section is made rostral to the midbrain, rigidity is no longer present and all the components of the righting reflexes, as described below, are present. In these animals the distribution of muscular tone is normal, that is, tone is present in both flexor and extensor muscles, while in the decerebrate animal the tone is essentially extensor in character. The midbrain animal cannot only maintain the four-legged standing posture, but can also rise to standing ("right itself") if overthrown, which the decerebrate animal cannot do.

The reactions of the midbrain animal are most conveniently studied if the cut is made rostral to the thalamus, in which case the animal's heat-regulating mechanism is functioning.

An analysis of the righting function of the midbrain and the thalamus animals disclosed that five groups of reflexes were involved. Each of these five groups of reflexes were studied separately in cats, dogs, and monkeys by reducing the animal to the so-called "zero condition." This condition obtains if the blindfolded animal, following bilateral labyrinthectomy, is held freely in the air without touching the ground. Under these conditions no righting reflexes can be evoked, and the animal is completely disoriented.

LABYRINTHINE-RIGHTING REFLEXES ACTING ON THE HEAD

These reflexes serve to orient the head in space. They are present in thalamus animals (cats, dogs, and monkeys) with intact labyrinths. The blindfolded animal is held by the pelvis in the air, and regardless of which position the pelvis is held in (laterally, obliquely, etc.), the head rights itself, that is, assumes a position that is normal for the animal. These reflexes originate in the labyrinths, as a result of the effect of gravity on the receptor organs in the labyrinths, and act primarily on the neck muscles. Destruction of the labyrinths abolishes the reflexes.

BODY-RIGHTING REFLEXES ACTING ON THE HEAD

If a "zero condition" animal is held freely in the air in the lateral position, the head remains in the lateral position. But if the animal is placed on its side on a table, the head rights itself. In this case the reflex is evoked by stimulation of afferent receptors on the side of the body that is in contact with the table. However, if a weighted board is placed on the upper side, the stimulus becomes bilateral, and the head falls back into the lateral position. When the board is taken away, the head again rights itself. This indicates that *asymmetrical body contact is the effective stimulus.*

In intact animals, the two above-mentioned reflexes both contribute to the righting of the animal's head.

NECK-RIGHTING REFLEXES
ACTING ON THE BODY

When the animal lies on its side and the head rights itself (as a result of either or both of the head-righting reflexes), the neck becomes twisted. Impulses set up by such twisting evokes another reflex which brings the upper portion of the animal's body in line with the head. This movement is accompanied by rotation in the lumbar region of the vertebral column which, in turn, evokes a reflex causing the hind portion of the body to align itself with the thorax and the head. This completes the righting of the entire body.

The author points out that the neck-righting reflexes make it possible for a man to throw a strong animal on its side by twisting its head.

BODY-RIGHTING REFLEXES
ACTING ON THE BODY

If the animal is placed on its side on the table and the head is held firmly in the lateral position, the animal's body tends to right itself in spite of the neck-righting reflexes, which tend to keep the body aligned with the head. The stimuli for the body-righting reflexes acting on the body arise from asymmetrical contact of the lateral side of the body with the supporting surface. This may be demonstrated by placing a weighted board on the uppermost lateral side of the body. With such bilateral stimulation, the body remains in the lateral position.

OPTIC-RIGHTING REFLEXES

It has previously been noted that reducing an animal to the "zero condition" includes blindfolding; such animals are disoriented in space and the head does not right itself. In normal animals of higher species (cats, dogs, monkeys) the eyes play a role in the righting of the head.

The optic-righting reflexes may be studied in animals whose labyrinths have been destroyed and who are held freely in the air. If the eyes are open and the animal's gaze becomes fixed on a familiar object, the head will right itself. If the visual attention ceases, the head is likely to return to its abnormal position.

The author assumes that the centers for the optic-righting reflexes are located in the optic cortex, but he states that he has no definite proof that this is the case.

CENTERS FOR THE RIGHTING REFLEXES

The centers for the righting reflexes (except for the optic reflexes) were determined by Rademaker (1926), an associate of Magnus. The neck-righting reflexes acting on the body were found to be located in the pontine region. The other three reflexes are said to have their seats in the ventral portion of the midbrain just in front of the third nerve. Rademaker had good reasons to believe that the red nuclei situated in this region harbor the centers for the labyrinthine reflexes acting on the head, and for the body-righting reflexes acting on the body, and that the efferent impulses for these reflexes are conducted in the rubrospinal tracts. The body-righting reflexes acting on the head were found to have their centers at the same level, but not in the red nuclei.

THE RED NUCLEI

In the thalamus animal, destruction of the red nuclei or severance of the rubrospinal tracts disrupts impulses that contribute to normal tone of flexor and extensor muscles, and decerebrate rigidity sets in. It may therefore be concluded that impulses conducted by the rubrospinal tracts serve to modify influences from lower centers (medulla and spinal cord), which are responsible for marked increase in tone of the extensor muscles and loss of tone of the flexor muscles.

In the intact animal, severance of the rubrospinal tracts has less severe effects than those in the thalamus animal. This finding leads to the conclusion that the cerebral cortex also contributes to the counterbalancing of influences from lower centers. If both the rubrospinal and the pyramidal tracts are severed, decerebrate rigidity becomes fully developed.

RIGHTING REFLEXES IN MAN

The nature of righting reflexes in man are less well known than in animals. Probably, the optic-righting reflexes are more important, and the labyrinthine reflexes less important in man than in animals.

As an example of the importance of optic-righting reflexes in man, the author cites the experience of aviators who become disoriented in space when flying through clouds. When they emerge from the clouds and can again see the ground, they may discover that they had completely misjudged their position with respect to the ground.

Landau (1925) and Schaltenbrand (1925) pointed out that head- and neck-righting reflexes are quite active in children. Infants in the prone position tend to bring the head into a normal position by dorsiflexion of the head and neck. Passive rotation of an infant's head in the supine position will cause the child to roll over to the lateral position. According to Zingerle (1925), the neck-righting reflex acting on the body can also be demonstrated in some patients.

REFERENCES

Landau, A. Ueber motorische Besonderheiten des zweiten Lebenshalbjahres. *Mschr. Kinderheilk.* 29:555, 1925.

Rademaker, G. G. J. *Die Bedeutung der roten Kerne und des übrigen Mittelhirns für Muskeltonus, Körperstellung und Labyrinthreflexe.* Berlin, Springer, 1926.

Schaltenbrand, G. Normale Bewegungs- und Haltungs- und Lagereaktionen bei Kindern. *Deutsch. Z. Nervenheilk.* 87:23, 1925.

Zingerle, H. Klinische Studien über Haltungs- und Stellreflexe, sowie andere automatische Körperbewegungen beim Menschen. *Z. Psychol. Neurol.* 31:330, 1925.

Abstract 16

R. Magnus, and A. de Kleijn

Die Abhängigkeit des Tonus der Extremitätenmuskeln von der Kopfstellung (The Influence of the Position of the Head on the Tone of the Muscles of the Extremities)

Pflüger Arch. Physiol. **145**:455–548, 1912

During previous studies on decerebrate cats, an influence of the position of the head on the tone of the extremities had been observed. It had been discovered by chance that if the animal's head posture was altered, a change in tone* of the muscles of the limbs resulted. But a specific head movement was accompanied by different reactions depending upon the body posture of the animal. The authors could find no obvious reasons for the varied reactions.

The present study was undertaken at the Pharmacological Institute, Reichsuniversität, Utrecht, Holland, in an attempt to determine the rules governing the limb reactions. It took 3 years (90 experiments, over 1,000 observations) before the rules for the reactions could be formulated. Thirty of these experiments were conducted by Magnus, the remaining 60 by Magnus and de Kleijn jointly. The reflexes reported on are known as Magnus' and de Kleijn's reflexes.

The studies revealed that two types of influences were present, one originating in the neck (tonic neck reflex), the other in the labyrinths (tonic labyrinthine reflex). It was demonstrated that these two types of reflexes are present in intact animals, but for the present study decerebrate preparations had to be used in order to prevent influences from

* *Remarks by S. Brunnstrom:* The term *tone* (Tonus) as used by the authors refers to a reflex contraction in skeletal muscles. Such tone may be responsible for maintaining a limb in a specific position against an opposing force, such as gravity; changes in tone may cause increase or decrease in rigidity and may result in involuntary movements of the limbs.

higher centers from mixing with the reflexes. To determine in what manner the two types of reflexes—neck and labyrinthine—contribute to the motor outcome, each type was studied separately, which required that the other type be eliminated.

Decerebration of the type employed in this study results in marked increase in tension of the extensor muscles of the neck, back, tail, and limbs ("decerebrate rigidity," see Sherrington, Abstract 18). In such a preparation, the effects of the tonic neck and tonic labyrinthine reflexes are revealed by an increase or decrease in extensor rigidity of the limbs; simultaneously, the flexor muscles of the limbs are adversely affected because of the mechanism of reciprocal innervation.

For the investigation of tonic changes in the *forelimbs*, Sherrington's method of decerebration was used, consisting of section of the brainstem in the intercollicular region, combined with severance of the spinal cord in the lower thoracic region. This method, Sherrington had found, provides a preparation that is free of shock and responsive to stimuli. Severance of the spinal cord results in maximal reflex effects in the forelimbs and eliminates disturbances from the hind portion of the body. When the behavior of the *hindlimbs* was investigated, decerebrate animals with intact spinal cord were used.

STUDY OF THE TONIC NECK REFLEXES

The labyrinthine influences were permanently eliminated by severance of the eighth cranial nerve, or by extirpation of the labyrinth, or temporarily blocked by injection of a cocaine solution. The three methods gave the same results. The effects of bilateral and unilateral procedures were observed.

With labyrinthine influences absent bilaterally, movements of the head with respect to the trunk consistently evoked specific reactions, regardless of the animal's posture. The results were observed with the animal in the supine, prone, and side-lying positions, with the animal held suspended, head up or down, and with the animal placed in the standing position, maintained in that position because of the presence of extensor rigidity of the limbs.

The investigators distinguish between two types of neck reflexes: those elicited by *asymmetrical* head movements (rotation, side bending), and those evoked by *symmetrical* head movements (dorsiflexion, ventroflexion).

ASYMMETRICAL NECK REFLEXES

Head rotation and head side bending proved to have the same type of effect, but as a rule the response was less vivid when evoked by side bending than by rotation. Head rotation to the right increased the tone of the extensor muscles of fore- and hindlimbs on the right side; it simultaneously decreased the tone of the extensor muscles of the fore- and hindlimbs on the left side. Head rotation to the left had the opposite effects. The rules governing these responses are expressed as *extension of the jaw limbs, flexion of the skull limbs,* the "jaw limbs" being those limbs toward which the animal's snout is turned, the "skull limbs" those limbs toward which the back of the animal's head is turned. The asymmetrical neck reflexes thus produce opposite responses of the limbs on the right and on the left sides.

SYMMETRICAL NECK REFLEXES

Dorsiflexion of the head and neck increases the tension in the extensor muscles of both forelimbs and decreases the tone of the extensor muscles of both hindlimbs. Ventroflexion of the head and neck has the opposite effect, that is, it decreases the tone in the extensor muscles of both forelimbs and increases the

tone of the extensor muscles of both hindlimbs. Thus, the effect of these reflexes is symmetrical, but fore- and hindlimbs respond in opposite directions. The rules for the symmetrical neck reflexes may be expressed as follows: *Dorsiflexion of the head results in extension of the forelimbs and flexion of the hindlimbs; ventroflexion of the head results in flexion of the forelimbs and extension of the hindlimbs.* These reflexes, as a rule, were found to have less marked effects than those of the asymmetrical reflexes.

VERTEBRA PROMINENS REFLEX

If pressure is applied in a ventral direction to the vertebral column in the region of the seventh cervical and the first thoracic vertebrae, all four limbs flex. The vertebra prominens reflex must be distinguished from the reflexes evoked by dorsiflexion and ventroflexion of the head and neck.

Evidence is presented in support of the view that the centers for the tonic neck reflexes are located in the upper two or three cervical segments of the spinal cord. After the posterior roots of C1, C2, and C3 had been severed bilaterally, the neck reflexes, except for the vertebra prominens reflex, were no longer obtained. The question of whether tonic neck reflexes originate from proprioceptors in the muscles, or in the joints, of the cervical spine was not determined by the authors.*

STUDY OF TONIC LABYRINTHINE REFLEXES

A plaster jacket was applied to the animal's head, neck, and upper trunk in such a manner that neither symmetrical nor asymmetrical head-neck movements could take place. This

* *Remarks by S. Brunnstrom:* A more recent study by other investigators led to the conclusion that receptors in the joints of the upper portion of the neck, especially the atlanto-occipital and atlanto-axial joints, were chiefly responsible for the neck reflexes. This conclusion was drawn because neck reflexes were still present after afferent impulses from neck muscles had been eliminated. (McCouch, G. P., Deering, I. D., and Ling, T. H. Location of receptors for tonic neck reflexes. *J. Neurophysiol.* 14:191–195, 1951.)

procedure permitted the authors to study the effects of the tonic labyrinthine reflexes without interference from the neck reflexes.

The labyrinthine reflexes originate in the otolith organs of the inner ear. These organs are not influenced by movements of the head and neck unless the head alters its position with respect to the horizontal plane; nor are they influenced by pure translatory movements of the head. These reflexes cause an increase or decrease of the tone of the extensor muscles of the limbs as a result of *specific positions of the head in space.*

The labyrinthine reflexes act identically on the muscles of all four limbs. There is one position in space which produces maximal extensor tone of the limb muscles and one position which produces minimum extensor tone, and these two positions are 180 degrees apart. In most of the experiments the *extensor tone was maximal when the animal's abdomen was up and its mouth cleft was 45 degrees above the horizontal plane; the extensor tone was minimal after the animal had been rotated 180 degrees about a horizontal axis.* In all other positions of the head, intermedial values of extensor tone was obtained. Figure 1 illustrates the manner in which the position of the

animal's head in space affects the tone of the muscles of the limbs.

Frames of a motion picture taken during one of the experiments are reproduced in Figure 2, showing the cat in a plaster jacket with rubber bands slung around the neck and around the paws. When the animal's position was changed from that of minimal extensor tone to that of maximal extensor tone, the forelimbs extended against the force of gravity and the resistance by the rubber bands. The extensor response occurred slowly and was preceded by a latency of several seconds. Once maximal extensor tone had been developed, it persisted for a long period of time. It appeared as if the muscular reaction was nonfatiguing.

Other experiments on decerebrate cats demonstrated that the influence of the midbrain as well as that of the cerebellum could be eliminated without causing a disturbance of the labyrinthine reflex. These and additional experiments led to the conclusion that the centers for the labyrinthine reflexes lie caudally to the entrance of the eighth nerve into the medulla. Experiments further showed that *one intact labyrinth suffices to evoke bilateral reflex activity.*

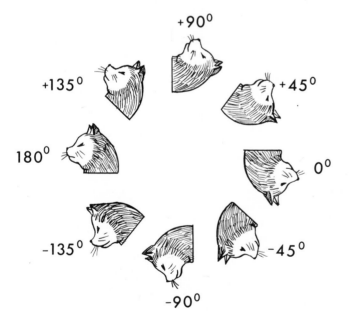

FIGURE 1. Scheme for head positions in the investigation of tonic labyrinthine reflexes in decerebrate cat. Maximal extensor tension in the limbs develops when the mouth cleft stands 45 degrees above the horizontal at +45 degrees. Minimal extensor tone is found at −135 degrees. (Redrawn from Magnus and de Kleijn, Die Abhängigkeit des Tonus der Extremitätenmuskeln von der Kopfstellung. *Pflüger Arch. Physiol.* 145:455–548, 1912.)

SELECTED ADDITIONAL COMMENTS BY THE AUTHORS

Both labyrinthine and neck reflexes are attitudinal reflexes; they last as long as the head position in question is maintained. The reflex effects were observed to persist as long as one hour.

The reflex effects are most marked at shoulder and hip, elbow and knee. Ankle and toe joints participate to a lesser extent.

The outcome of the combined reflexes can always be explained as the arithmetic summation of neck and labyrinthine reflexes, regardless of the posture of the animal.

In the animals examined, the latency of the labyrinthine reflexes varied between ⅓ and 23 seconds; that of the neck reflexes, between ⅓ and 6 seconds.

Experiments with dogs demonstrate that, generally, the same reflexes are present in dogs as in cats.

It was also shown that the above-mentioned reflexes exert an influence on movements of animals with intact nervous systems.

Evidence is presented that tonic neck reflexes are present also in human subjects when, for pathological reasons, certain impulses from the cerebral hemispheres are more or less eliminated. The reflexes in man follow the same rules as those established for animals. Labyrinthine reflexes in man, the authors state, are also probably present, but these reflexes had not been confirmed with certainty by the authors.

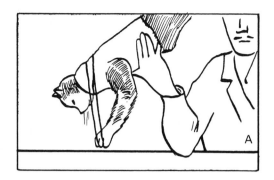

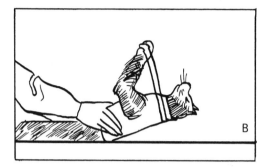

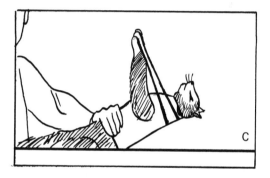

FIGURE 2. Frames from a motion picture illustrating labyrinthine reflexes in decerebrate cat. The reflexes are elicited by changing the position of the animal's head in space. The tonic neck reflexes have been eliminated by the application of a plaster jacket, which prevents head and neck movements. (Redrawn from Magnus and de Kleijn, Die Abhängigkeit des Tonus der Extremitätenmuskeln von der Kopfstellung. *Pflüger Arch. Physiol.* 145:455–548, 1912.) *A.* At starting position, extensor tone is minimal. The forepaws are pulled toward the neck by rubber bands. *B.* The animal has been turned around 180 degrees to the position of maximal extensor tone. No change in the tone of the forelimbs is noticed immediately. *C.* About 5 seconds later the limbs have extended against the resistance of the rubber bands and maximal extensor tone has developed.

Abstract 17

P. Marie and C. Foix

Les Syncinésies des Hémiplégiques (Synkinesis in Hemiplegia)

Rev. Neurol. 29:3–27 and 30:145–162, 1916

Pierre Marie, well-known French neurologist who was Chief of the Neurological Service, La Salpetrière Hospital, Paris, devoted much time to the study and interpretation of the motor behavior of patients with hemiplegia.

The publication reported here was co-authored by Charles Foix, an associate of Marie, and consists of two parts. Part I deals with terms and classification of synkinetic phenomena and contains a review and a criticism of the interpretation of these phenomena by other authors. In Part II, the physiology and pathology of motor disturbances in hemiplegia are discussed from a theoretical and a practical standpoint.

The term *synkinesis*, the authors state, was coined by Vulpian, a Parisian physician (1826–1887), and has since been employed by authors and clinicians to mean involuntary movements and movement combinations evoked by muscular activity, usually voluntary, in some part of the body.

The synkinetic phenomena observed by Marie and Foix are classified under three headings: *global synkinesis, imitation synkinesis,* and *coordination synkinesis.*

GLOBAL SYNKINESIS

Global or spastic synkinesis ("la syncinésie globale où spasmodique") manifests itself as a generalized tenseness of the muscles on the affected side. If the patient performs a movement on the normal side—any movement—and his effort is strong, the limbs on the affected side begin to move and assume attitudes that do not vary in an individual patient; they can be evoked with regularity.

In general, these attitudes are exaggerations of muscular contractures already present, that is, flexion contracture of the upper limb and extension contracture of the lower limb. However, patients were also observed who responded with extension of the upper limb and, more rarely, flexion of the lower limb.

IMITATION SYNKINESIS

Imitation synkinesis was found to be less common than global synkinesis. The authors postulate that imitation synkinesis is related to the normal difficulty of performing different (asymmetrical) movements on the two sides of the body. Symmetrical movements are always easier to perform. The "mirror image" movements described by Meige are such facilitated movements.

Patients who display imitation synkinesis probably attempt to facilitate the execution of a difficult movement by performing the identical movement on the other side. True imitation synkinesis is observed on the *normal side*. As an example, when the patient attempts, perhaps without success, to move the fingers on the affected side, it may be observed that the fingers on the normal side perform that same movement. The patient is unaware of the imitation movements, but if his attention is drawn to them they can easily be inhibited by will.

The abduction and adduction phenomena described by Raimiste are symmetrical and identical movements of the two lower limbs, and may at first glance be taken for imitation synkinesis. However, these phenomena have little in common with true imitation synkinesis and, in the opinion of the authors, should be classified as coordination synkinesis.

COORDINATION SYNKINESIS

Two types of coordination synkinesis are observed in the lower limb, namely, a shortening synkinesis ("syncinésie de raccourcissment") and a lengthening synkinesis ("syncinésie d'allongement").

The *shortening synkinesis* of the lower limb consists of flexion at hip, knee, and ankle. A patient with hemiplegia in the supine position who is asked to dorsiflex the foot at the ankle may be unable to do so. But a voluntary flexion of the hip is accompanied by an automatic dorsiflexion of the ankle. This ankle movement also appears if the patient makes an effort to flex the hip while the investigator prevents hip flexion by firm resistance. Thus a joint movement is performed synkinetically while it cannot be initiated by voluntary effort. The synkinetic movements are inseparably linked to each other and all efforts at separation are useless.

The *lengthening synkinesis* of the lower limb manifests itself as a total elongation of the limb. For example, when a patient is asked to extend the knee, an involuntary plantar flexion of the ankle appears. The patient is unable to perform the ankle movement in an isolated fashion; if he attempts to do so, the quadriceps muscles contract synkinetically. It is pointed out that the tendency to contract the quadriceps muscles when plantar flexion is willed is present also in normal persons. In hemiplegia, this tendency is exaggerated and cannot be overcome.

Coordination synkinesis in the *upper limb* presents more variations than in the lower limb. Usually, voluntary elevation of the shoulder girdle is accompanied by abduction at the shoulder, and voluntary depression of the shoulder girdle by synkinetic adduction of the arm. It was also observed that when a patient flexes the elbow by voluntary effort the fingers also flex; this may be a manifestation of a shortening synkinesis, the authors state, but it may also be a result of a global synkinesis. Coordination synkinesis is responsible for a patient's inability to move one of the digits in an isolated fashion; if he attempts to do so, all fingers move together. This is simply an exaggeration of a normal tendency.

The question raised as to whether or not the *finger phenomenon of Souques* should be regarded as a component of the lengthening synkinesis of the upper limb, but this question is left unanswered. (Souques observed that in some, but not all patients with hemiplegia, an elevation of the arm overhead is accompanied by an automatic extension of the fingers.)

The authors believe that synkinetic phenomena have diagnostic value. Whereas the presence of spinal reflexes indicates that the spinal cord is functioning, the presence of synkinetic movements indicates that nervous centers located on levels higher than the spinal cord are participating. For diagnostic purposes, a table of tests to be used for the investigation of synkinetic phenomena is presented. This table, labeled "gymnastique syncinétique," is found at the end of Part II of the original publication. There is no mention, however, of the use of the table as a guide for therapeutic exercise, as may erroneously be assumed from the word "gymnastique."

Abstract 18

C. S. Sherrington

Decerebrate Rigidity and Reflex Coordination of Movement

J. Physiol. 22:319–332, 1898

This is a report on the result of experimental decerebration (ablation of the cerebral hemispheres) in monkeys, dogs, cats, rabbits, and guinea pigs, animals that all react in essentially the same manner.

Whereas section through the upper portion of the spinal cord or through the lower portion of the medulla results in muscular flaccidity, the condition following decerebration is characterized by rigidity. When an animal with bulbar section is held in the air, its limbs hang limply in the postures imposed on them by gravity. In contrast, the limbs of the decerebrate animal are held stiff in extension. The condition is described as follows:

"It [the monkey] hangs with its forelimbs thrust backward, with retraction at the shoulder joint, straightened elbow, and some flexion at wrist. The hand of the monkey is turned with its palmar face somewhat inward. The hindlimbs are similarly kept straightened and thrust backward; the hip is extended, the knee very stiffly extended, and the ankle somewhat extended. The tail in spite of its own weight, and it is quite heavy in some species of monkeys, it kept either straight and horizontal or often curved upward. . . . The head is kept lifted against gravity and the chin is tilted upward under the retraction and backward rotation of the skull."

In the monkey, as well as in other animals, the forelimbs are more rigid than the hindlimbs. The knees and elbows are markedly stiff, while wrist and ankles are less affected.

Following bilateral decerebration, rigidity usually develops after a few minutes. In some animals it may persist as long as 4 hours. Rigidity is less marked after ablation of only one hemisphere; rigidity then develops mainly on the *homolateral* side.

If the posterior nerve roots in the cervical region are severed on one side while decerebrate rigidity is present, the forelimb on that side immediately becomes flaccid. Deafferentation of the lower limb has the same effect. If the posterior roots are severed some days prior to decerebration, rigidity may not develop at all, or develops poorly. This indicates that afferent impulses from the limbs are essential for the development and maintenance of decerebrate rigidity.

The decerebrate preparation may be utilized for studying of inhibitory impulses arising in the central nervous system, or peripherally. Various tracts in the spinal cord and certain areas of the brain, as well as peripheral nerves and skin, were stimulated electrically or by other means, and the effects observed. From these and other studies, principles governing reflex coordination of movement, notably the principle of *reciprocal innervation of antagonistic muscles*, were derived.

Remarks by S. Brunnstrom: In this publication, decerebrate rigidity resulting from "ablation of the cerebral hemispheres" is discussed. The caudal and rostral limits for transections which produce decerebrate rigidity were more accurately determined at a later date. In 1910, Sherrington (see Abstract 20) defined the decerebrate preparation as "one in which the whole brain in front of the posterior colliculi has been removed."

Abstract 19

C. S. Sherrington

The Integrative Action of the Nervous System

New Haven, Yale University Press, 1906
2nd edition, 1947, Reprinted 1961

In this valuable book, now a classic, Sherrington has assembled a wealth of information concerning the function of the nervous system. Information was derived from laboratory experiments on higher mammals such as dogs and cats. The integration of nerve cells, nerve conduction pathways, and specific mechanisms by means of which an individual can function as a coordinated whole is elucidated.

Throughout this book (as well as in the author's many individual research reports), the interrelation between sensory input and motor responses is stressed. The all-important role of reflex activity in integration is discussed. For therapists who are presently employing various types of sensory stimulation in an attempt to enhance motor function, Sherrington's work offers invaluable guidance.

Certain portions of this book are here briefly reviewed for the benefit of those readers who are not already well informed. To attempt a comprehensive abstract of the book here is out of the question; the original should be consulted frequently by all rehabilitation personnel interested in neurophysiology.

REFLEXES

Reflexes supply the foundation of the integrative action of the nervous system. In Sherrington's words, *"The unit reaction of nervous integration is the reflex,* because every reflex is an integrative reaction, and no nervous action short of a reflex is a complete act of integration. . . . Coordination, therefore, is in part the compounding of reflexes" (p. 7).

"TYPE-REFLEXES"

Among the type-reflexes studied by the author may be mentioned the *flexion reflex* and the *crossed extension reflex*. These two reflexes exhibit motor responses consisting of gross flexion and gross extension and are characterized by reciprocal innervation of antagonistic muscle groups.

In a type-reflex the neural arcs of the components are interconnected in the spinal cord to "something of a unitary mechanism." Furthermore, "the elements seem incapable of isolated excitation" (p. 78). However, one component of a type-reflex may respond alone to a very weak stimulus; but if the intensity of the stimulus is increased, the other components will follow. This is an example of *irradiation*.

Irradiation may occur not only between components of a type-reflex, but may spread to other functionally related reflexes. For example, if the stimulus which evokes a flexion reflex of the hindlimb of a spinal dog be gradually intensified, the contralateral hindlimb will extend ("crossed extension"), then the ipsilateral forelimb will extend, and the contralateral forelimb will flex (p. 153).

The *extensor thrust* (pp. 67–69, 90) is an ipsilateral spinal cord reflex, evoked by pressure on the plantar surface of the dog's hindfoot, or by inserting a fingertip between the plantar cushion and the toe pads, causing a spreading of the pads. The reflex is well marked in the spinal dog in which even light stroking of the skin behind the plantar cushion may suffice to evoke a response. Such response is more likely to materialize if, prior to the stimulus, the knee and hip are passively placed in flexion.

The motor response consists of a momentary strong extension of hip, knee, and ankle. Simultaneously, the antagonistic flexor muscles are inhibited. The duration of this response, the author found, was usually about one fifth of a second (Fig. 1). But the succeeding refractory period, during which time the reflex cannot be elicited, was quite long, often lasting six times as long as the active response.

Sherrington observed that in the spinal dog the extensor thrust was powerful enough to raise the animal's entire body from the ground and push it forward. This and other evidence caused him to conclude that the extensor thrust had evolved to supply the force required during the propulsion phase of animal locomotion. Its use in locomotion would explain the length of the refractory period because, after push-off, considerable time is required for the limb to flex and swing forward in preparation for the next step.*

* *Remarks by S. Brunnstrom:* In treating adult patients with spastic hemiplegia, this reviewer has never observed an extensor response of as short duration as that characterizing the extensor thrust. In hemiplegia, the extensor response is comparatively sustained and is accompanied by co-con-

SUCCESSIVE REFLEXES

Reflexes that proceed simultaneously must be coordinated not only among themselves, but also with those reflexes that proceed successively. The latter coordination is achieved by means of a spinal mechanism referred to as *successive induction.*

Figure 2 illustrates the myograph curves of the crossed extension reflex evoked by electrical stimuli applied to the contralateral foot at regular intervals (once a minute). If the repetitive stimuli are weak but of constant intensity and duration, the muscular responses are weak (as seen in *A*) and uniform throughout.

In the experiment illustrated, the crossed extension reflex *B* became markedly intensified with respect both to amplitude and duration when in the interval between *A* and *B* a flexion reflex was evoked on the same side and maintained for 55 seconds. The influence of the flexion reflex (which was intercalated between *A* and *B*) on reflexes *C, D,* and *E*

traction of the flexor muscles, which is not true of the extensor thrust. If Sherrington's nomenclature is honored, the term *extensor thrust* is a misnomer when applied to neuromuscular extensor responses in patients with hemiplegia.

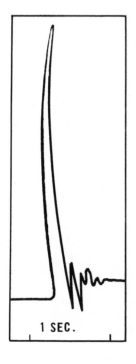

FIGURE 1. The extensor thrust in spinal dog. The application of the stimulus is not indicated, but the latency is very brief. (Redrawn from Sherrington, C. S. *The Integrative Action of the Nervous System,* 2nd ed. New Haven, Yale Univ. Press, 1947, p. 67.)

1 SEC.

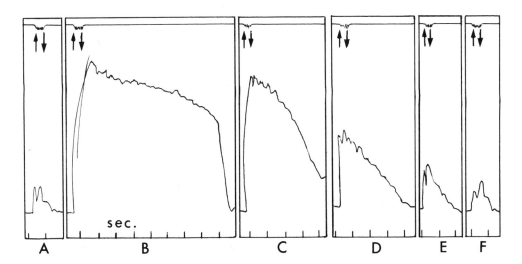

FIGURE 2. Successive induction. The crossed extension reflex of the hindlimb of a dog is augmented by a precurrent flexion reflex (see text). (Redrawn from Sherrington, C. S. *The Integrative Action of the Nervous System,* 2nd ed. New Haven, Yale Univ. Press, 1947, p. 209.)

was a gradually declining one. In *F*, the reflex has assumed its original shape (as in *A*). "Now as we have seen, *during* the flexion reflex the extensor arcs were inhibited: *after* the flexion reflex these arcs are evidently in a phase of exalted excitability" (p. 208).

Under certain conditions, the exalted excita-

bility of a reflex arc as a result of a precurrent antagonistic reflex may reach such proportions that the reflex appears spontaneously immediately following the cessation of the stimulus which evoked the antagonistic reflex. In that case, reflex stepping movements of a spinal animal may appear, because each successive reflex excites the neural arcs of the other.

This review has covered only selected aspects of reflex action of the spinal cord dealt with in the first six chapters of Sherrington's book. In subsequent chapters, reflexes as adapted reactions, some aspects of the reactions of the motor cortex, dominance of the brain, and sensual fusion are discussed.

Abstract 20

C. S. Sherrington

Flexion Reflex of the Limb, Crossed Extension Reflex and Reflex Stepping in Standing

J. Physiol. 40:28–121, 1910

The most readily evoked skin reflex in spinal dog, cat, and frog is flexion. It can be elicited in both the upper and lower limb by stimulation of the skin, or of an afferent nerve. The reflex consists of flexion at hip, knee, and ankle in the lower limb, and of flexion at shoulder, elbow, and wrist in the upper limb. This spinal reflex can easily be elicited also in the decerebrate preparation; it is commonly referred to as the "flexion reflex of Sherrington."

If the reflex is evoked by a painful stimulus, its effectiveness increases and it becomes dominant in competition with other reflexes, that is, it may interrupt another reflex already in progress. This powerful reflex is referred to as the "nociceptive flexion reflex."

In the preliminary investigation, decerebrate preparations were used and the reflex was evoked from a cutaneous nerve branch close to the annular ligament of the ankle. The nerve was severed and its proximal stump tied. The stump was stimulated either with faradic current, or mechanically, by tightening a loop of thread previously slung around the stump.

When the reflex was evoked in this manner, certain muscles responded regularly. The reflex did not spread to other limb muscles, no matter how intense the stimulus. The muscles which participate in the flexion reflex of the lower limb are listed in Table 1.

Since in the decerebrate preparation a considerable tension is present in the extensor

Remarks by S. Brunnstrom: The term "tensor fasciae femoris" was used by anatomists when this publication appeared. "Tensor fasciae latae" became the approved term at a later date.

TABLE 1

Ilio-psoas	Semitendinosus
Pectineus (weak response)	Biceps femoris posterior
Sartorius (portion of)	Tenuissimus
Tensor fasciae femoris* (weak response)	Tibialis anticus
	Peroneus longus (variable)
Rectus femoris	Extensor longus
Gracilis	digitorum

muscles of the limb, the inhibitory effect of the flexion reflex on these muscles may also be studied. The muscles which are inhibited by the flexion reflex are listed in Table 2.

Increase in intensity of the stimulus did not cause the inhibition to spread to additional muscles, but it intensified the inhibitory effect on the muscles listed in Table 2. The muscles inhibited by the flexion reflex are the same muscles which are activated in the crossed extension reflex.

Sherrington's report is accompanied by an illustration which schematically shows the muscular arrangement in the lower limb of the

TABLE 2

Vastus lateralis	Biceps femoris anterior
Vastus medialis	
Crureus	Flexor longus digitorum(?)
Gastrocnemius	
Soleus	Quadratus femoris
Semimembranosus	Adductor minor
	Adductor magnus (portion of)

cat. For example, the semitendinosus muscle, in cat as in man, originates above the hip joint and inserts below the knee joint. Its action as a knee flexor by far exceeds its action as a hip extensor. It contracts during the flexion reflex and has a low threshold of excitation.

The semimembranosus muscle in the cat originates above the hip and inserts on the lower end of the femur, hence it has no direct action on the knee. In spite of its proximity to the semitendinosus muscle, it does not become excited during the flexion reflex, even when a very strong stimulus is employed. On the contrary, it becomes *inhibited*, and thus belongs to the extensor muscles.

The biceps femoris in the cat consists of two separate muscles with different functions. Both muscles originate on the pelvis. The biceps femoris posterior inserts on the tibia halfway down the leg. It flexes the knee and extends the hip and, like the semitendinosus, is more of a knee flexor than a hip extensor. It is excited in the flexion reflex. The biceps femoris anterior is inserted near the knee joint, mainly on the femur, and is a hip extensor. It is inhibited by the flexion reflex.

By applying the stimulus on the animal's lower limb from the toes all the way up to the groin in front and the ischial region in back, the author determined that the flexion reflex could be evoked anywhere within this area (the "receptive field"). The threshold was lowest distally, particularly on the toe pads and on the plantar cushion; in general, it rose gradually as the stimulating electrode was placed more proximally. A high threshold, however, was found in the region of the calf muscles.

Although the reflex could be evoked from an adequate stimulus throughout the receptive field, the reflex results varied somewhat, inasmuch as the response of certain muscles varied in strength, depending upon the point of stimulation. A detailed report of these variations is supplied. The general characteristics of the reflex, however, did not change.

When the stimulus was applied to one or the other of the cutaneous nerves supplying the skin near or above the border line of the receptive field, the reflex would change from flexion to extension.

It is pointed out that the receptive field of the flexion reflex is "not merely an area of surface, a skin-field, but is musculo-articular as well, and includes the whole thickness of the limb as well as its surface. In this respect the receptive field of the flexion reflex differs fundamentally from a receptive field such as that of the scratch reflex which is wholly cutaneous."

The studies of the flexion reflex and its accompanying crossed extension reflex in decerebrate, and in spinal preparations, proved that these reactions are governed by the principle of *reciprocal innervation of antagonistic muscles*. This principle applied to flexor and extensor muscles of the various joints. However, there was co-contraction of antagonistic rotary components, such as those supplied by the semitendinosus and the biceps femoris posterior muscles.

Remarks by S. Brunnstrom: The above material is abstracted from Section I of Sherrington's 1910 report. Additional sections discuss reflex movements accessory to the flexion reflex, reflex standing, and reflex walking. These sections supply a wealth of information and are well worth a careful study.

Abstract 21

A. Simons

Kopfhaltung und Muskeltonus (Head Posture and Muscle Tone)

Z. Neurol.* 80:499–549, 1923

This is a detailed report on a clinical investigation of associated reaction in patients with hemiplegia. In the years 1916–1918, Simons observed these reactions on brain-injured patients who were casualties of World War I. The investigation was later extended to patients with other types of neurologic disorders, children as well as adults. It soon became evident that two types of patients were best suited for the investigation: (1) adult patients with hemiplegia, whether caused by trauma, tumor, or cerebral vascular accident, and (2) children with cerebral palsy.

The author collected data on 248 patients, most of whom were examined repeatedly on different days according to a standardized testing procedure. The patients' reactions were observed with the patient supine, sitting, standing, and walking.

A convenient method of evoking associated reactions, the author states, is to have the patient clench the fist on the normal side. This stimulus usually sufficed to evoke a reaction, but occasionally reinforcement was required, such as resistance to a movement on the unaffected side, clenching of the jaws, or contraction of the abdominal muscles. If a strong muscular contraction on the unaffected side proved ineffective, an effort to move the affected lower limb would at times result in marked response of the affected upper limb.

Ordinarily, a considerable effort on the part of the patient was required for the reaction to materialize, but in exceptional cases a very mild stimulus sufficed. In one patient with hemiplegia the closing of the eyelid on the

normal side elicited vivid associated movements on the affected side; in another patient an imaginary clenching of the fist brought results.

The associated reactions did not always result in joint movement but often manifested themselves only as changes in tension in the various muscle groups. When this was the case, resistance to passive movements was tested to assess such changes.

An influence of the head position on the pattern of the associated movement was first observed by the author in 1916. Figure 1 illustrates a typical case. The patient had suffered a brain injury from a gunshot two months previously and exhibited vigorous associated movements, the patterns of which were regularly reversed when the examiner rotated the patient's head from one side to the other. Following this discovery, and throughout this lengthy study, the investigator paid close attention to the effect of head positioning. He came to the conclusion that the phenomena were manifestations of the tonic neck reflexes, as described by Magnus and de Kleijn (see Abstract 16). However, since the associated movements did not materialize on passive head movements as observed in animals, he assumed that reinforcement was required for the neck reflexes to become observable; such reinforcement was supplied by the patient's voluntary muscular contractions elsewhere in the body.

The data collected by Simons indicated that, in general, the associated movements followed the rules for the asymmetrical neck reflexes in animals ("flexion of the skull limbs, extension of the jaw limbs"). The influence of lateral inclination of the head was observable,

* Formerly *Zschr. f.d.g. Neurol. u. Psychiat.*

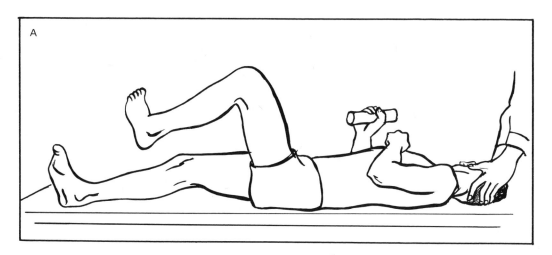

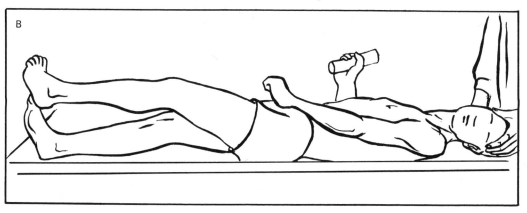

FIGURE 1. Patient with left-sided hemiparesis following a gunshot injury during World War I. *A.* With the head rotated toward the right, a typical flexor synergy of the lower limb developed. The elbow flexed and the fist closed. *B.* With the head rotated to the left, extensor synergies appeared in both upper and lower limbs. (Redrawn from frames of a motion picture, from Simons, A. Kopfhaltung und Muskeltonus. *Z. Neurol. 80:*499, 1923.)

but less clearly than that of head rotation. Ventroflexion and dorsiflexion of the head did not always evoke symmetrical neck reflexes in the same manner as in animals. In fact, the effect was often opposite in direction.

In a comparatively small number of patients with hemiplegia atypical and irregular reactions were observed which the author was unable to explain.

The latency period of the reactions varied among patients. At times an associated movement developed as soon as the muscles on the normal side contracted, at other times a latency of several seconds was present. In some patients, the latency period often varied from one examination to the other. The upper and the lower limbs frequently had different latencies. The sequence of joint movements was inconsistent; at times all segments of the limb started to move simultaneously, while at other times a step-by-step activation of the various segments was observed.

In a limited number of patients electromyography was used to study the behavior of the biceps and the triceps brachii muscles. On some days, a typical action current of the agonist was present with simultaneous inhibition of the antagonist; on other days, without any changes in the testing procedure having been made, the same patient exhibited co-contraction of the two muscle pairs.

Simons was aware that in man, as in animal, tonic labyrinthine reflexes may, at least in part, be responsible for the change in muscle tone in the extremities. His clinical findings indicate, however, that in human subjects the neck reflexes predominate over the labyrinthine reflexes.

Simons' original article is accompanied by 12 plates of photographs of patients exhibiting associated reactions.

T. Tokizane, M. Murao, T. Ogata, and T. Kendo

Electromyographic Studies of Tonic Neck, Lumbar, and Labyrynthine Reflexes in Normal Persons

Jap. J. Physiol. 2:130–146, 1951

The rules for the tonic neck and labyrinthine reflexes of Magnus and de Kleijn are reviewed.

The tonic lumbar reflexes were discovered by two Japanese investigators, Shimamoto and Nakajima, and reported in a Japanese journal in 1943 and 1944 (text in Japanese language). These reflexes are evoked by changes in the position of the upper part of the body with respect to the pelvis. The investigation was conducted on decerebrate rabbits, cats, and dogs. The tone of the muscles of the limbs is said to be affected in the following manner:

Rotation of the trunk to the right evoked flexion of the right forelimb, extension of the right hindlimb. Simultaneously, the left forelimb extended and the left hindlimb flexed. Trunk rotation toward the left had the opposite effect on all limbs.

Lateral flexion of the trunk was found to have the same effect as trunk rotation—that is, flexion of the forelimb and extension of the hindlimb on the side toward which the trunk deviated.

Trunk movements in anteroposterior directions had different effects in rabbits than in cats and dogs. In the rabbit, dorsiflexion evoked extension of all four limbs, ventroflexion flexion of all four limbs. In cats and dogs, dorsiflexion of the trunk caused flexion of both forelimbs, extension of both hindlimbs. Ventroflexion had the opposite effect.

The present study is concerned with the effect of tonic neck, lumbar, and labyrinthine reflexes in adult human subjects, as revealed by electromyography. Six subjects participated: four normal men, one normal woman, and one deaf-mute individual whose labyrinthine function was completely abolished.

The changes in the electrical activity of the muscles were recorded with needle electrodes. Because it was desirable to record both facilitatory and inhibitory influences, the subjects learned to maintain a constant weak voluntary contraction in the muscles being examined. In the presence of a weak muscular contraction, it becomes possible to identify spike discharges of a single neuromuscular unit with a fairly uniform discharge interval in the electromyogram. Superimposition of a weak reflex effect results in a shortening of the discharge interval when a facilitatory effect is present, in a lengthening of the discharge interval when an inhibitory effect is present.

The ensuing changes in the discharge intervals were graded and recorded by using a scale of plus signs (+, + +, + + +) and minus signs (−, − −, − − −). Variable effects were indicated by a plus-minus sign (±), and no effects by a zero sign (0).

TONIC NECK REFLEXES

The subject was seated and the position of his head was passively changed at a slow rate. The effects on the electromyograms of the following head positions were investigated: rotation toward the left, side-bending to the left, rotation to the right, side-bending to the right, dorsiflexion, and ventroflexion. A detailed account of the electromyographic findings for selected muscles of the upper and lower limbs, resulting from the six different head positions, are given in table form. As an example, head rotation toward the left had the following effects on the muscles of the limbs on the left side:

Deltoid	+
Triceps brachii	+ + +
Wrist extensors	0
Wrist flexors	0
Gluteus maximus	+
Vastus medialis	+ +
Vastus lateralis	+ +
Biceps femoris, long head	+
Gastrocnemius	+
Soleus	+ +
Tibialis anterior	−

The deaf-mute subject displayed the same effects of the tonic neck reflexes as did the other five subjects.

The authors do not state which portion of the deltoid muscle was sampled, but this reviewer assumes that it was the anterior portion, which may possibly associate itself with the extensor muscles (pectoralis major, triceps). The long head of the biceps femoris was also linked to the extensor muscles, apparently as a hip-extensor muscle,* and, not surprisingly, so were the calf muscles. The response was quite marked in the elbow muscles, while no effect was detected in the wrist muscles.

Since the neck reflexes have a *tonic* influence, it is quite logical that the effect on the soleus muscle, a predominantly "red" muscle which passes one joint only, should be more marked than on the gastrocnemius, a two-joint muscle, the fibers of which are predominantly of the "pale" type. For the same reason, there was more response in the medial and lateral heads of the triceps, which are one-joint muscles, than on the long head of the triceps, a two-joint muscle.

The symmetrical tonic neck reflexes were found to have the same effect in the experimental subjects as in animals. Dorsiflexion of the head had a bilateral facilitatory effect on the extensor muscles of the upper limbs; ventroflexion had the opposite effect. The responses in the ankle muscles were inconsistent (±).

THE TONIC LUMBAR REFLEXES

The subjects were seated or assumed the supine position on a table. The examiner passively moved the trunk by rotation, side-bending, flexion, or extension. To prevent evoking neck reflexes, a corset was applied over the neck which prevented neck movements. The effects observed in the electromyograms could thus be attributed to lumbar reflexes without interference by neck reflexes.

In each trunk position, facilitation and inhibition of the electrical activities of the muscles conformed to effects obtained in animal experiments. Responses were observed in both upper and lower limbs; they were most marked in the lower limbs. In general, the reflex effects were less pronounced than those evoked by neck movements. The deaf-mute subject responded in the same manner as the other subjects.

The results are set forth in detail in table form (Table II of the original article), excerpts of which are given below. When the trunk was rotated toward the left, the muscles on the left side responded as follows:

Deltoid	0
Triceps brachii	−
Biceps brachii	+
Wrist extensors	0
Wrist flexors	0
Gluteus maximus	+
Vastus medialis	+ +
Vastus lateralis	+ +
Biceps femoris, long head	+
Gastrocnemius	±
Soleus	±
Tibialis anterior	±

TONIC LABYRINTHINE REFLEXES

The subject to be examined was strapped to a revolving table in the prone or supine position in such a manner that no changes could take place in the joints of the neck and the limbs. The table was slowly rotated 360 degrees about a frontal axis and the changes in the electromyograms observed. In general, the responses in the normal subjects con-

---

* *Remarks by S. Brunnstrom:* Note that in the cat the "biceps femoris anterior" originates above the hip joint and inserts into the femur just above the knee joint (see Sherrington, Abstract 20). It extends the hip and may, indirectly, also extend the knee, because of its traction on the femur in a posterior direction.

formed with those obtained in animal experiments (see Magnus and de Kleijn, Abstract 16). The deaf-mute subject displayed no effect whatsoever from changes in the position of the head in space.

Thus, it was demonstrated that effects of the tonic neck, lumbar, and labyrinthine reflexes were present in normal subjects. These effects were quite weak as compared to those observed in decerebrate animals, in normal infants, and in patients with certain neurological disorders.

Abstract 23

T. E. Twitchell

The Restoration of Motor Function Following Hemiplegia in Man

Brain 74:443–480, 1951

The sequence of motor recovery of 121 patients with hemiplegia was investigated at Boston City Hospital. These patients, with the exception of three, were diagnosed as cerebral vascular accidents caused by thrombosis or embolus of one of the cerebral vessels. At the time the report was written, no autopsy results were available, hence the exact location of the lesion could not be determined. Each patient was examined at regular intervals, and electromyographic records were obtained from some of the patients. The motor recovery of both upper and lower limbs were observed, but attention was focused on the upper limb, in particular on the course of restoration of the grasping function of the hand. Slight sensory defects were found present in 87 of the 121 patients.

An analysis of the data collected in this study indicated that the recovery process followed a general pattern. There was a remarkable uniformity in the sequences of recovery of all patients. This was true regardless of whether sensory disturbances were present and whether the dominant or nondominant hemisphere was involved. The patients progressed from one recovery phase to the next in an orderly fashion without any of the phases being omitted. The same sequence was followed by patients who recovered completely as well as by those patients whose recovery was arrested at any one of the stages.

Immediately following the cerebral vascular accident, the condition was essentially flaccid, with loss or hypoactivity of the tendon reflexes. Thereafter, the following recovery phases were observed:

1. The finger jerks could be elicited.

2. Spasticity—that is, resistance to passive movements—appeared.
3. Proprioceptive facilitation was obtained; reflexes and willed movements were mutually facilitatory.
4. Proximal traction response was present (traction on one group of flexor muscles of the upper limb evoked responses of all flexors of that limb).
5. Some voluntary hand movements were performed without proprioceptive facilitation.
6. Tactile stimuli of the palm of the hand facilitated and/or reinforced the grasp.
7. A true grasp reflex could be elicited (see Seyffarth and Denny-Brown, 1948).
8. Recovery became complete.*

Twenty-five patients were followed until a comparatively stable condition had been reached. In this group were five patients who recovered fully, even though the upper limb of these patients had been completely paralyzed at the onset. These patients passed through each one of the stages outlined above in a comparatively short period of time. Stage 7 (the grasp reflex) was reached in 23 to 40 days. Thereafter, 20 to 40 additional days were required for full recovery.

From a prognostic standpoint, the time required for arriving at Stages 3 and 4 was considered significant. Those patients who recovered completely reached these stages in 10 days or less; a longer period of time (15

---

* Recovery was considered complete when movements could be performed as skillfully and as speedily on the affected side as on the normal side. At this time, blindfolding did not adversely affect movements.

to 46 days) was required for patients whose recovery was incomplete and for those who never progressed beyond the flexor synergy of the upper limb. The patients who failed to respond to proprioceptive facilitation did not recover any willed movements whatsoever. In general, the longer the duration of the flaccid period, the poorer the prognosis.

Spasticity when first observed was mild in all patients. In patients who were on their way to good or full recovery, spasticity reached its peak in 10 to 18 days and never became severe. The less fortunate patients displayed an increase in intensity of spasticity for a longer period of time, and many developed severe spasticity. Such prolonged spasticity indicated that the prognosis for restoration of motor function was unfavorable.

The flexor synergy of the upper limb was the first movement pattern to recover and was generally followed by an extensor synergy. However, in some patients the recovery of the upper limb was limited to the flexor synergy, and the extensor synergy did not appear. In the lower limb return of flexion also preceded extension, but later, extension predominated.

Flexion of the fingers was first obtained as a part of the total flexor synergy. The fingers could not be flexed in an isolated manner until much later (if recovery continued). During the spastic period of recovery proprioceptive stimuli were most effective as facilitatory agents. As spasticity declined and some voluntary hand movements appeared, tactile stimuli were found instrumental in developing a more complete hand function. The true grasp reflex, evoked by a distally moving tactile stimulus in the palm of the hand, always preceded full recovery. Coordinated hand movements evolved gradually by modification of elementary proprioceptive and contactual responses. When the grasp reflex failed to appear, recovery remained incomplete.

In both upper and lower limbs the synergies of flexion and extension developed before isolated movements of the various joints could be mastered. The author points out that, in general, primitive responses constitute the bases from which more elaborate responses and movements evolve.

The tonic neck reflex (evoked by forceful active head rotation) was found to decrease spasticity in one of the upper limbs, in accordance with the rules formulated by Magnus and de Kleijn. The influence of the body-righting reflexes was also well observable. When the patient was lying on his side with the affected limbs on the upper side, flexion of elbow, wrist, and fingers increased; lying on the other side—with the affected limbs on the lower side—had the opposite effect. In the former position, a proximal traction response was obtained in those patients who exhibited hyperactive proprioceptive reactions. In the latter position flexor tension diminished and some extension appeared.

As long as spasticity prevailed, a certain latency of voluntary motor responses was observed, and relaxation following a contraction was slow. For example, a latent period of 2 to 5 seconds was present between the time a command for a movement was given and the time the movement began; relaxation of contraction required 1 to 3 seconds. When a patient attempted to reverse a movement from flexion to extension this could only be done by allowing a brief pause at the turning point. All willed movements were performed slowly and fatigued easily. At this time, the elimination of vision increased the motor defect.

In summary, motor recovery following hemiplegia began with a simple proprioceptive reaction, the stretch reflex; thereafter, more complex proprioceptive reactions, such as the proximal traction response, evolved; next, the patient learned to utilize the limb synergies—first the flexor synergy, then the extensor synergy. All proprioceptive responses were influenced by neck- and body-righting reflexes. As spasticity declined, willed movements improved and these could be facilitated and modified by tactile stimuli. Tactile stimuli played a continued role in the development of coordinated hand function.

The author concludes:

"The course of recovery from cerebral paralysis does not favour the division of motor function into separate independent entities such as segmental reflexes, neck reflexes, labyrinthine and body-righting reflexes and optic-righting reflexes. Each of the more complex members of these is composed of elements of the less complex. The ability for willed movement is therefore not a separate and indivisible function. The present study indicates the part played by these factors in the course of recovery from hemiplegia, and provides a rationale for proprioceptive and contactual exercises in the re-training of movement."

REFERENCE

Seyffarth, H., and Denny-Brown, D. The grasp reflex and the instinctive grasp reaction. *Brain* 71:109, 1948.

Abstract 24

T. E. Twitchell

Sensory Factors of Purposive Movement

J. Neurophysiol. 17:239–252, 1854

Previous investigators, notably Mott and Sherrington (1895), had found that depriving a monkey of all sensation in one upper limb by posterior rhizotomy resulted in an almost complete paralysis of that limb. The limb was not used for walking, running, climbing, or grasping food. However, very little motor deficiency was observed if a portion of the cutaneous sensation in the hand was intact, even when the afferent muscle nerves were severed.

The above-mentioned experiments by Mott and Sherrington were repeated by Twitchell who wished to make his own observations in an attempt to analyze the neuromuscular mechanisms responsible for the return of certain types of motor activity following total or partial deafferentation of one upper limb in monkeys.

RESULTS

COMPLETE DEAFFERENTATION

The posterior roots of C3 through T3 were severed, depriving the animal of all sensation in the upper limb. In general, the findings of the previous investigators were substantiated.

Immediately after surgery and for several days thereafter, the limb was functionally paralyzed, although occasionally some uncontrolled associated movements of flexion and extension were observed, particularly when the animal was excited. A few days after the operation the animal began to ward off painful stimuli (such as pin-pricks) with a gross, poorly coordinated flexion movement of wrist and elbow in an attempt to catch the insulting object and pull it toward the mouth. At a later date, an extension movement was also observed as the animal tried to push an annoying object away. Strong motivation was required to evoke these two defensive motor acts which had to be guided by vision and which could only be used in a limited area on the ventral side of the body. The arm was not used for running, climbing, grooming, or feeding. The ability to use the hand for grasping was permanently lost. The animal was seen chewing on the deafferented limb and precautions had to be taken to prevent him from chewing it off.

It was observed that the above gross movements were related to, and dependent upon, the position of the animal's head with respect to the trunk. The head was markedly ventroflexed during the flexor movement. The posture during the push-away movement was characterized by arching of the back and some dorsiflexion of the head. Head rotation was also seen accompanying flexion or extension movements. The author suspected that the movements observed were neck reflexes which the animal was able to adapt for purposes of defense. After the tonic neck reflexes had been abolished by section of the uppermost cervical roots bilaterally, no movements of the deafferented limb were observed. The limb hung flaccidly and the hand dragged on the ground when the animal moved around. The author's conclusions were thus substantiated.

PRESERVATION OF ONE CUTANEOUS DERMATOME

When one sensory root supplying a portion of the hand was spared, the animal used the limb in a near normal manner for walking, climbing, feeding, and grooming. The grasping function of the hand was quite good, but the grasp was weaker than normal. Some ataxia and overreaching was observed as the animal reached out to grasp an object, but these defects disappeared in about 2 weeks, having apparently been compensated for by vision.

If one sensory root supplying the skin of the upper arm was spared (C5 or T2), all other roots being sectioned, no sensation in the hand remained and much more motor defect resulted. Immediately following operation, the motor behavior of these animals closely resembled that of animals with total deafferentation. The limb was not used for moving around, for grasping, or for defense from pin-prick.

After a considerable time—6 weeks to 2 months or longer—a certain amount of function returned, more rapidly in the C5 animal than in the T2 animal. The limb was used occasionally for walking and running and eventually for grasping. The animal learned to defend itself when teased with a pin by using a gross flexion or extension movement. In both the C5 and the T2 animal movements had to be directed by vision.

In the C5 animal, grasp was observed only in conjunction with flexion of wrist, elbow, and shoulder, that is, as a component of the total flexor synergy. This reaction, the author observes, closely resembles the proximal traction response characteristic of the spastic stage of human patients with hemiplegia (see Twitchell, Abstract 23).

The T2 animal also learned to grasp, but utilized a different neuromuscular mechanism.

The proximal traction response was absent. Because T2 also distributes to the finger flexor muscles, the grasp in the T2 animal was believed to have resulted from interaction between the tonic neck reflex and the local stretch reflex, which mechanism the animal was able to adapt to purposeful activity.

This research report contains a wealth of information useful to rehabilitation personnel and deserves to be read in its entirety. In the discussion at the end of the report the following points are stressed:

1. Interruption of the sensory portion of the sensorimotor mechanism results in far greater motor deficit than a lesion in the Rolanic motor area or of the pyramidal tracts (see Denny-Brown, Abstract 3). Without sensation, the limb is practically useless, even though motor areas and motor pathways for the upper limb are intact.
2. Both exteroceptive and proprioceptive impulses are highly important for motor function.
3. The preservation of cutaneous sensation in the hand is indispensable for motor function of the upper limb.
4. Movements of the upper limb, and in particular the grasping function of the hand, is directed by contactual stimuli.

REFERENCE

Mott, F. W., and Sherrington, C. S. Experiments upon the influence of sensory nerves upon movement and nutrition of the limbs. Preliminary communication. *Proc. Roy. Soc.* 57:481, 1895.

Abstract 25

J. von Uexküll

Studien Ueber den Tonus II. Die Bewegungen der Schlangensterne (Muscle Tone Studies II. The Movements of the Brittlestar)

Z. Biol. 46:1–37, 1905

An experiment with Ophioglyphia Lacertosa, an animal belonging to the starfish family, is described.

Five long, round, and very mobile arms protrude from the central portion of the animal's body which contains the digestive organs. An osseous ring enclosing the central part of the animal's nervous system encircles the mouth. The innervation to the muscles of the arm comes from the nerve centers inside the bony ring.

For the study of the laws that govern the movements of this simple animal, a portion of the central body is dissected away so that only the osseous ring containing the nerve structures is retained. Four of the five arms are carefully removed. The osseous ring is then severed at a point opposite the remaining arm, which disrupts the continuity of the nerve ring. The preparation is attached to a cork slab mounted on a tripod. The slab can be rotated to allow the preparation to hang with the arm completely vertical, or in the manner illustrated in Figure 1.

If the arm is hanging vertically without any bend at the root of the arm and the point R^I is stimulated electrically, the arm responds with a swing toward the side of R^I. If stimulated at R^{II}, the response is toward that side. But if the animal's position is such as illustrated in Figure 1, the response is always toward the side of R^I, regardless of whether the stimulus is applied at R^I or R^{II}.

This and other studies by von Uexküll indicate that the peripheral muscles are instrumental in determining the path of the impulses arising from the electrical stimulation. The fundamental law applicable to the conduction of nerve impulses in a simple nerve net is expressed as follows:

The impulses always flow toward the elongated muscles (Es fliesst die Erregung immer zu den verlängerten Muskeln).

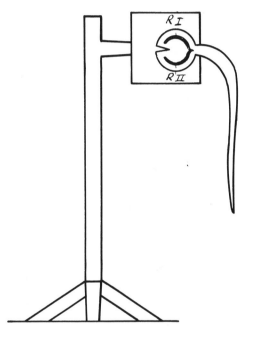

FIGURE 1. Von Uexküll's arrangement for demonstrating effect of elongation of muscles on reflex responses (see text). (Redrawn from von Uexküll, Studien über den Tonus II. Die Bewegungen der Schlangensterne. **Z. Biol.** **46:1–37, 1905.**)

Remark by S. Brunnstrom: This rule came to be known as the von Uexküll-Magnus' rule (see Magnus, Abstracts 12 and 13).

Index

Author Index

Page numbers in *italics* refer to illustrations

Subject Index

Page numbers in *italics* refer to illustrations